LONG LIVE THE 12 RULES TO LIVE LONG

A NATURAL HEALTHY LIFE

BY JORDAN RIVER

Introduction

When it comes to getting older, we all want to age gracefully and happily. But, at the same time, almost all of us strive to accomplish this; very few people know how to achieve it. So, what is the real deal? Is it proper nutrition, exercise, and involvement? The brief answer is 'Yes,' but it actually amounts to a lot more. In fact, the secret to a healthy and long life lies in our lifestyle and environment.

The concept is somewhat easy to understand, but not many people know how it works. What we eat and drink, the company we keep, and our willingness to take risks in life will dictate how long we live. Believe it or not, there are ways around increasing your chances of getting old gracefully. And yet when you think about these things, they are all life choices. These rules can keep you looking youthful, feeling young and healthy for a long time to come—a real possibility if practiced daily, consistently.

Throughout my life experiences, I have realized that there are 12 essential rules to live a long and fulfilling life. This book talks about all those magical rules briefly and how each rule has the potential of transforming your life positively.

As you would have already guessed, the first rule talks about the importance of a healthy diet in our lives. What we eat defines how we feel and look, affecting our moods. Eating healthy is essential to living a long life. When we eat the right things, we can avoid diseases such as diabetes, hypertension, obesity, or others that damage us from the inside.

The second and third rules talk about the usage of certain herbs and drinks to boost our intake of nutrients every day. Since water is the ultimate elixir of life, it is the most essential drink that our body requires. However, the book also lays great emphasis on other drinks that impact the quality of our lives in multiple ways.

The fourth rule focuses on family, society, and how important it is to be with your loved ones in life. It is no secret that we all want to lead a life full of love and affection. We can all attest to the fact that when we feel loved and cared for, we tend to live longer and happier lives.

The fifth rule talks about sleep and its importance in our lifestyle. The book discusses how much sleep we actually need each day and how to ensure that we get the right amount of sleep even while working. We all know that, in our busy lives, it is not always possible to get 8-9 hours of sleep each night. However, you might not know that there are other methods to help you fall asleep easily and quickly.

The sixth rule deals with the importance of exercise in our lives. You might be wondering how much you should exercise in your day-to-day life. I have already told you that when you eat healthily, sleep well, and drink the right things; it becomes difficult to make time to work out. But from someone who has 'been there and done that', I know exercise is the secret to a long life.

The seventh rule focuses on mental wellness and how it is an essential part of our lives. The book explores different aspects of maintaining mental health, what they are, and why you should care about them. It also talks about how one can maintain their mental health through yoga or meditation daily.

The eighth rule ties in with the seventh one. It talks about the importance of maintaining a healthy lifestyle and explains why it is important to consistently practice certain things.

Lifestyle is something that people have little control over because you don't really get to choose what kind of family or society you are born into. However, a positive and healthy lifestyle is something that we can decide for ourselves. It talks about different aspects of being healthy, from what you eat to how much you sleep.

The ninth rule delves into our jobs and how it impacts our health as well as the quality of our lives. For example, working too hard without any breaks or just not taking care of ourselves in the workplace can result in accidents or minor health issues that go unnoticed.

The tenth rule talks about passion and how it is one of the most essential things in your life. It is said that when you do what you love to do, you never feel like working because you are always engrossed in doing something that you love.

However, jobs and money are necessary to survive in today's world. So, what is the solution? The right approach is to have a creative outlet and devote time to it!

The eleventh rule talks about spirituality and its importance in our lives. Living a long life is not just about eating healthy or working out. It also involves being comfortable in your skin and being at peace with yourself and the world around you. Spirituality helps us connect with the universe and lets us enjoy life more than we might otherwise do.

The final rule is the most important of them all. It talks about dopamine detox and its benefits in our lives. Dopamine is a chemical that regulates mood, sleep, and feelings of happiness.

Most people are unaware that they have an addiction to dopamine because their brains are used to being constantly stimulated by it. The problem with dopamine is that it can cause us to focus on meaningless things instead of having more meaningful experiences.

It talks about how dopamine detox will help you get through the withdrawal phase by helping you deal with your cravings for dopamine in a more healthy way. It also suggests ways in which one can make their life healthier and happier, both physically and mentally.

The 12 rules in the book may seem like a lot to follow, but they will make you healthier and happier if appropriately followed. They can also help you to live a longer life. Isn't that our primary goal? So let's learn more about each of these rules in detail and make them a part of our lives. Are you ready?

Chapter 1: Live a long life with a healthy diet

Don't we all visualize ourselves aging gracefully and living a long, healthy, and happy life? While many people associate a long life with an individual's genes, science says otherwise. According to research performed on 3000 pairs of DNAs of identical twins who later adopted different lifestyle choices, only 25% of their longevity was attributed to their genes. Instead, a whopping 75% was affected by the lifestyle choices made by them. Clearly, our lifespan is influenced by the lifestyle we choose for ourselves.

We all have different dreams and desires about our bodies and overall health. For example, some of us want to lose weight, improve our health, or boost our athletic ability. But how many of us pay attention to the food we eat or the overall diet that we provide to our body? Very few!

Your daily diet can either add many healthy years to your life or take years off your life expectancy. It is one of the most important factors influencing how long you will live. A balanced, nutritious-packed diet supplies your body with all the essential ingredients it requires to function at its full potential. A healthy lifestyle diet, which includes regular physical activity and avoiding harmful substances like smoking and alcohol, can add many healthy years to your life expectancy. On the other hand, an unbalanced or unhealthy lifestyle diet will result in obesity, diabetes, heart diseases, etc., thus shortening your lifespan.

Even the holy book Hindu, Bhagavad Gita, recites the importance of the type of food one should consume. It puts forth three types of food; Sattvic, Rajasic, Tamasic. Satvic refers to the ideal date for a human, Rajasic to greedy eating, and Tamasic to ignorant eating. Sattvic food, hence, emphasizes the easily digestible food good for the important organs. These kinds of food, as per the book, increase the lifespan and make you stronger. Hence, it is not me telling you, but the way life should be, to watch what you eat. Doesn't that signify how vital a well-balanced diet is?

What is a balanced diet?

A balanced diet is one that includes all the essential nutrients required by the body, such as carbohydrates, proteins, vitamins, minerals, and other micronutrients. A balanced diet will ensure that your body gets all the essential ingredients it needs to function at its full potential and stay healthy and happy.

What should be included in a balanced diet?

The body requires twelve different nutrients. The amount of each nutrient your daily diet should include is already decided upon by many health professionals and nutritionists around the world. However, the recommended daily allowance (RDA) for these nutrients differs according to age, gender, weight, height, level of physical activity, etc., so you must consult your physician to know what you should include in your balanced diet.

The following information illustrates the components of a healthy, balanced diet:

Carbohydrates (45-65%)

Carbohydrates provide energy to the body and are present in different forms such as starches, sugars, dietary fibers, etc. Carbohydrates can be subdivided into sugars, starches, and dietary fibers. A healthy diet should include more complex carbohydrates than simple carbs. Complex carbohydrate sources are those that contain high levels of fiber, such as whole grains, veggies, legumes, etc., while simple carbohydrates are found in sugary foods like candies, etc.

Fats (20%)

Healthy fats are required by the body to keep cells healthy, protect organs, and also aid in insulation. However, there are two types of fats: saturated fat and unsaturated fat. One must include monounsaturated or polyunsaturated fat sources in their daily food regimen since they lower cholesterol levels, prevent blood clots, reduce inflammation, etc. Foods like nuts, avocados, olives, olive oil, canola oil, flax seeds, etc., are good sources of monounsaturated fats. In addition, whole foods like unhulled sesame seeds and soybeans contain polyunsaturated fat sources.

Vitamins (5%)

Vitamins A, C, and E are antioxidants that prevent or slow down degenerative diseases like cancer. Vitamin C also aids in the absorption of iron. Broccoli, strawberries, citrus fruits, etc., all contain high levels of vitamin C, while carrots and tomatoes are excellent sources of vitamin A.

Protein (10%)

The body requires protein to build bones, muscles, cartilage, and other tissues. Protein is necessary for growth as well as to maintain muscle mass. Therefore, one must include protein-rich foods such as lean meat, fish, legumes, etc., in their diet daily as they promote optimum health and improve the overall quality of life.

How to ensure the consumption of a balanced diet?

1. Vegetables (3-5 servings)

Most physicians around the world recommend that you include five servings of vegetables and fruits in your daily diet. Fruits and vegetables are good sources of vitamins, minerals, and other micronutrients that keep your body healthy and fit. Even the Quran, the holy book of Muslims, emphasizes the need for a balanced diet containing ample vegetables, fruits, and salad, in its verse 6.99. It encourages moderation in eating and avoiding extravagant portions. That's why I give attention to servings, and you should follow the same. Vegetables especially contain phytochemicals, which provide a vast array of health benefits such as cancer prevention etc.

Amongst veggies, asparagus is one of the most nutritious of all. In fact, science has it that this vegetable (which looks like spinal cord) the decellularized asparagus plant tissue can be used to grow or regenerate the living bodily tissues. The same has been proven by an experiment done by Dr. Pelling on rats under which he found that integrating asparagus scaffolding to the rat tissues actually reversed the problem of severed spinal cords. In fact, many rats were able to walk again.

Imagine the benefits that regular consumption of this vegetable can bring to your body!

2. Water (1 fluid ounce per 1 kilo of your weight. So a person who weighs about 200 pounds should drink about 1 gallon of water per day)

It is important that you drink the adequate amount of water daily to keep your body hydrated, to aid in digestion, and to also help eliminate toxins. Water also balances the pH levels in your body and maintains electrolyte balance. You can include green tea, black tea, herbal tea, etc., as they are good sources of antioxidants like catechins, flavonoids, etc.

3. Calcium (1-2 servings)

Calcium is required to keep bones healthy and strong. Therefore, one must include calcium-rich foods in their diet. Some of these are dairy products like milk, cheese, yogurt, etc., green leafy veggies like turnip greens, broccoli, soybeans, etc., calcium-fortified products like orange juice, cereals, etc., almonds, sesame seeds, etc.

4. Fatty Acids (2-3 servings)

Fatty acids are used in the body to produce energy. There are two types of fatty acid: saturated fat and unsaturated fat. A healthy diet should include three servings of unsaturated fat sources like fish, flax seeds, etc., every week since they lower cholesterol levels and keep your heart healthy.

5. Iron (30-40mg)

Iron is required to carry oxygen in the blood cells. Therefore, it is vital that you have adequate amounts of iron to prevent anemia which often results from a deficiency of iron. Iron-rich food sources are green leafy veggies, lentils, beans, etc., so include them in your diet if you do not have enough iron-rich foods.

6. Protein (50-60g)

A healthy diet should contain at least 50-60gms of protein daily. Protein is required to build muscles, cells, and tissues. Pork, beef, chicken, fish are great sources of protein, so include them in your daily food regimen. If you are looking for vegan or vegetarian food items to get the required proteins, you can use soy products like tofu, soy milk, etc., in your diet.

7. Zinc (15mg)

Zinc is required to keep your immune system healthy and strong. Foods like seafood, meat, beans, etc., are good sources of zinc, so include these in your daily food regimen. You can also take supplements if you cannot include zinc-rich foods in your daily diet.

Foods to Avoid

1. Sugar (limit its consumption): High sugar diets are unhealthy since they cause insulin resistance and increased risk of diabetes and cardiovascular diseases. Excess intake of sugar also results in tooth decay,

obesity, etc. Hence one should include less sugar in their daily recipes. Salt (limit its consumption)

2. Salt: Excess salt intake causes high blood pressure, heart problems, and water retention. It is recommended that you cut back on salty food items like pickles and processed foods and consume less than 2gms of sodium daily.

3. Processed Food: One must altogether avoid processed food items as they contain refined sugar, high fructose corn syrup, trans fat, etc. Avoid taking processed meats as they may contain nitrates which are carcinogenic in nature.

4. Alcohol: Excessive alcohol intake causes liver diseases, heart problems, obesity, and cancer. It is advised to limit your daily intake of alcohol to one serving.

5. Tobacco: Tobacco smoking is terrible for the lungs as it results in respiratory ailments like lung cancer etc. Avoid smoking as much as you can.

Healthy food items to include in your daily diet:

1. Whole grains: Whole grains like oats, brown rice, barley, wheat bread, etc., should be a major part of your diet since they help improve heart health and lower the risk of diabetes and cardiovascular diseases.

2. Fruits: Blueberries can help heart health, bone strength, skin health, blood pressure, diabetes management, cancer prevention, and mental health. One cup of blueberries provides 24 percent of a person's recommended daily allowance of vitamin C. Fruits like apples, bananas, oranges, grapes, etc., are great sources of vitamins, minerals, and antioxidants. They help keep your skin glowing and prevent you from contracting several types of cancer.

3. Veggies: Vegetables contain a high amount of fiber, which helps prevent digestive diseases and maintains healthy blood sugar levels. They are good sources of vitamins and minerals like calcium, iron, magnesium, etc.

4. Nuts and seeds: Nuts and seeds like pecans, peanuts, almonds, etc., are a great source of healthy fats. They also contain high amounts of fiber, protein, antioxidants, and minerals, which help fight inflammation and prevent several types of cancer.

5. Lean proteins: Chickpeas, lentils, beans, etc., are a great source of protein for vegetarians and also contain high amounts of fiber, antioxidants, and minerals. They help prevent several diseases which are caused due to inflammation.

Benefits of a healthy diet:

A healthy diet brings with it many benefits. Let us take a look at some of those benefits and the scientific evidence behind them:

1. Heart health: A healthy diet keeps your heart healthy since it helps in lowering cholesterol and blood pressure. It also keeps you free from several types of cancer that are caused due to high sugar diets like breast, colorectal cancers, etc. According to some sources, a diet rich in fruits and vegetables, along with increased exercise and healthful eating, may help you prevent up to 80% of early heart disease and stroke cases.

2. Reduced risk of cancer: A healthy diet rich in fruits and vegetables reduces your risk of certain types of cancer. Fruits and veggies contain antioxidants that help fight free radicals, a dangerous form of substances that can cause damage to cells in the body. According to some studies, people who eat at least five servings of fresh produce a day have a reduced risk of developing cancer as compared to those who eat less than one glass.

3. Weight loss: A healthy diet helps with weight loss as it contains low amounts of sugar and high amounts of fiber which help reduce body fat. A few studies suggest that a lower-calorie and higher-fiber diet may help obese individuals lose weight faster than restricting calorie intake alone. According to some experts, a South

Beach Diet where you consume whole grains and lean protein can help promote healthy weight loss.

4. Reduced risk of kidney stones: A diet rich in vegetables and fruits is known to increase the pH level of your urine, which helps prevent kidney stone formation. The increased intake of water keeps you hydrated and flushes out toxins from your body.

5. Better sleep: If you consume a lot of carbs at night, then it will cause disturbed sleep patterns and insomnia. If you want a good sleep, then it is recommended to have a high-protein diet before going to bed as it boosts your metabolism and helps with healthy weight loss. Do not eat 4 to 5 hours before bedtime. Digestion is the most taxing power use of the human body. When it takes a break, it starts cleaning out damaged cells and starts to burn stores of fat.

6. Healthy skin: A diet rich in fruits, veggies, and whole grains can help prevent acne breakouts by increasing blood circulation, which reduces excess sebum production. It also protects against UV radiation that can cause damage to the skin.

7. Healthy aging: A healthy diet keeps your heart healthy, reduces inflammation in the body, and also helps you stay mentally sharp. It may help prevent several chronic diseases like Alzheimer's disease, dementia, etc., which are caused due to old age.

8. Strong immune system: Processed foods are the root cause behind several diseases like obesity, diabetes, cardiovascular problems, etc. Hence it is advised that you stay away from processed food items. Eating healthy regularizes insulin levels and improves digestion which helps in maintaining a strong immune system. Hence it is advised to include healthy food items which are rich in proteins, minerals, and fiber.

9. Depression: It has been scientifically proven that low levels of omega-3 fatty acids increase the risk of depression since they help regulate moods. Therefore one should include oily fish like salmon, mackerel, etc., in their diet on a daily basis.

10. Longevity: Adopting a healthy lifestyle of not smoking, regular exercise, and eating healthy food can increase your lifespan. It also helps you maintain your weight, which brings several other health benefits like heart diseases, diabetes, etc.

11. Improved gut health: A healthy diet helps maintain balanced gut flora. Probiotics or "good bacteria" help improve the digestive system and aid in absorbing nutrients from the food we consume.

12. Improved memory: A healthy diet rich in vegetables and fruits can help improve your memory. Fruits and veggies contain a vital molecule known as flavonoids

which have been shown to reduce the risk of dementia by boosting mental performance.

13. Improved mood: Healthy eating habits play a key role in mood regulation since a balanced diet helps the body produce enough serotonin, which improves your mood.

14. Better skin: A healthy diet rich in whole foods, fish, and vegetables can help improve your skin by improving its texture and color. Also, consuming oily fish like salmon twice a week will keep you hydrated from the inside out, which helps maintain average oil production, improving your skin condition.

15. Improve physical performance: A balanced diet consisting of carbohydrates, proteins, and fats is known to improve athletic performance. Protein intake helps repair muscles which increase stamina and endurance. Carbohydrates provide energy, while dietary fats help maintain body temperature during strenuous activities like playing sports.

16. Diabetes management: A healthy diet with the right amount of carbs, proteins, and fats can help manage diabetes. Fibers can slow down carbohydrate digestion which keeps blood sugar levels stable throughout the day.

Quick tips for a healthful diet:

Several tiny, beneficial changes can be made to your diet, including:

- Switching to water and herbal tea instead of soft drinks has numerous health benefits.

- Every week or two, cut your meat consumption in half.

- Fresh fruit and vegetables should make up at least half of each meal.

- Swapping cow's milk for plant-based milk

- Instead of juice, which is high in sugar and devoid of fiber, eating whole fruits instead of purees can help reduce the risk.

- Avoiding processed meats, which are high in salt and may boost the chance of colon cancer, is a good idea.

- Eating more lean protein, which you can easily find in eggs, tofu, fish, and nuts.

Healthy eating brings lots of benefits and can drastically improve the quality of life. However, in order to attain the desired bodily goals, including longevity, it is essential to pay attention to the first secret out of the two secrets that we will discuss in this book. In further chapters, we will take a look at the other secrets of a long and healthy life. Are you ready to explore them?

Chapter 2: The magic of healthy drinks

The oldest living person in the world is currently 120 years old. That's a magnificent level of longevity! If science is to be believed, humans can live up to the age of 150 years as well. If you are into the idea of longevity and good health, you have to accept the idea of a balanced diet and healthy nutrition.

In the previous chapter, we understood the importance of a well-balanced diet in enhancing one's life span. Through this chapter, you will learn about the importance of including healthy drinks in your daily diet and their contribution to adding longevity to your life.

What are healthy drinks?

The drinks that we intake daily and the beverages we consume form an important part of our diet. A healthy drink has health benefits and can be consumed without worrying about any ill effects such as gaining weight.

People usually define healthy drinks as liquids that provide us with nutrients and help in strengthening the immune system. The nutritional value of such drinks includes vitamins, minerals, enzymes, amino acids, antioxidants, and other phytochemicals (natural compounds found in plants). However, there is no hard and fast rule to define a healthy beverage; it differs from person to person based on their lifestyle and dietary choices.

How do healthy drinks add longevity to your life?

A healthy drink can do wonders for your health. It not only makes you feel refreshed but also helps in enhancing the body's immune system.

One of the major causes of illnesses is stress, which occurs when an individual is unable to manage their response to internal or external stimuli. Although certain drugs help counter the effect of stress and its side effects, they fail in creating a long-lasting effect and can even cause harm to our body in the process. A healthy drink not only counters the ill effects of stress by providing energy and nourishment; it also works as a stress reliever by calming your nerves and giving you instant relief from physical pain. Moreover, such drinks add longevity to life because they provide nutrients like vitamins, minerals, antioxidants, etc., which are essential for a healthy life.

Water: The elixir of life

Water forms the most important part of a healthy drink. Around 60% to 70% of your body weight is made up of water. Your brain's water content is 80% on average, which means that you need a sufficient amount of water to maintain the optimum functionality of your brain. Apart from boosting cognitive functions, it also helps fight stress and depression by soothing your nerves.

Water does not only help in quenching thirst but also plays an essential role in digestion by helping food travel through our digestive system faster. It also works as a detoxifying agent by flushing out impurities from the body cells, thus keeping toxins at bay and preventing diseases like headache, fatigue, intestinal disorders, etc.

Therefore, it is advised that one must drink 1 fluid ounce per 1 kilo body weight per day. However, this amount must be increased as and when you exercise or sweat more during summers.

Drinking water is the easiest and one of the most effective ways to add longevity to your life. Water has various health benefits such as weight loss, relief from constipation, piles, etc., and strengthening immunity by increasing blood circulation throughout the body. It also acts as a natural detoxifier that flushes out all the harmful toxins from your body and provides antioxidants like vitamin C & E that help in fighting free radicals (responsible for premature aging). Moreover, drinking plenty of water helps in improving metabolism and nourishing all parts of your body with adequate nutrients.

Top 10 healthy drinks that can add longevity to your life

The top 10 healthy drinks that can add longevity to your life are:

1. Coconut Water

Coconut water is among the most popular and healthiest drinks of all time because of its unique composition of electrolytes, amino acids, enzymes, vitamins, minerals, etc. Drinking coconut water can help you maintain optimum hydration levels by controlling your thirst pangs and keeping muscle cramps at bay. In addition, it provides relief from physical pain. It helps increase the concentration levels of an individual as it consists of many nutrients like magnesium and potassium that help in energy production within cells.

Coconut water can add longevity to your life with the numerous health benefits it offers. It replenishes the electrolytes lost due to dehydration and helps control many diseases. Hence, coconut water is a must for a healthy and disease-free life.

2. Apple Cider Vinegar

Apple cider vinegar can be defined as a type of vinegar that is made from freshly pressed apples. ACV has been used for centuries in Ayurveda to cure various medical conditions like weight loss, indigestion, thyroid problems, etc. In addition,

ACV helps reduce cholesterol levels due to its high concentration of pectin fiber that acts as a binder and helps bind fats and remove them from the body. In addition to this, Apple Cider Vinegar can add longevity to your life by maintaining the electrolyte balance within the body. It also contains potassium which is essential for maintaining normal blood pressure levels and helps increase endurance levels by delaying the onset of fatigue during physical activities.

3. Green Tea

Green tea is one of the most popular beverages around the world because of its numerous health benefits that help us lead a healthy life. Studies have shown that green tea can help in weight loss, reduce cholesterol levels, delay the aging process, etc. What makes green tea special is its high concentration of catechins, antioxidants that prevent cell damage by free radicals and thus prevent various ailments like cancer, heart diseases, etc. Apart from this, it also regulates blood sugar levels and has anti-aging properties since it protects our skin by neutralizing the effect of free radicals, which are produced due to environmental pollution.

Green tea is prepared by steaming the leaves of the Camellia Sinensis plant, which is then dried. Green tea consists of caffeine that causes increased alertness in an individual. Moreover, green tea also contains nutrients like catechins, polyphenols, L-theanine, caffeine, etc.

Green tea is very beneficial for health and also adds longevity to one's life. It acts as an antioxidant that helps in protecting your body cells from damage caused by free radicals. It also helps in increasing the concentration levels of an individual due to its caffeine content. Moreover, drinking two cups of green tea on a daily basis will help you maintain optimum hydration levels by controlling your thirst pangs and keeping muscle cramps at bay. In addition, it provides relief from physical pain and helps increase the concentration levels of an individual because it contains many nutrients like magnesium and potassium, which help in energy production within cells.

4. Watermelon Juice

Watermelon juice is an excellent example of a healthy drink that provides instant relief from physical pain and mental stress by hydrating your body cells and flushing out harmful toxins present in them. In addition, drinking watermelon juice regularly will improve the functioning of kidneys and help enhance immunity.

The health benefits of drinking watermelon juice include weight loss, reduction in cholesterol levels, relief from constipation, etc. Furthermore, watermelon juice is an excellent diuretic that helps in flushing out harmful toxins present in your body and provides relief from conditions like arthritis, obesity, hypertension, etc. In addition, drinking two cups of watermelon juice on a daily basis will provide relief from fatigue caused due to heatstroke.

5. Rooibos Tea

Rooibos tea is also known as red tea because its reddish-brown color is made from leaves of rooibos (Aspalathus linearis) plant native to South Africa. It consists of calcium, iron, zinc, vitamin E, etc., which make it beneficial for health and enhances one's life by adding longevity.

Some of the health benefits of Rooibos Tea include prevention of cancer, reduction in blood pressure levels, relief from asthma, diabetes, and much more. It also contains anti-aging properties that prevent the skin cells from being damaged by free radicals due to exposure to UV radiations, etc.

6. Carrot Juice

Carrot juice is an excellent source of vitamins A and K, which help in strengthening your muscles and bones. Not only this, but it also helps in improving the vision in an individual by protecting your eyesight by neutralizing the free radicals present in them. The health benefits of drinking carrot juice include relief from eczema, relief from diarrhea, weight loss, etc. Moreover, it acts as a multi-purpose solution for various health problems like constipation relief, purifying blood, etc.

7. Green Vegetable Juice

Green vegetable juice is among the best examples of healthy drinks that provide nourishment to an individual by flushing out all the harmful toxins from your body and providing antioxidants. It acts as a powerful detoxifier and helps in improving metabolism, which aids in weight loss. Moreover, it also provides relief from conditions like constipation, colitis, piles, etc., and strengthens immunity by increasing blood circulation throughout the body.

8. Red Grape Juice

Red grapes are known for their refreshing taste and high nutritional benefits due to their unique composition of nutrients like vitamins A & C, lycopene, pectin fiber, etc. In addition, it has various health benefits such as weight loss, relief from constipation, piles, etc., and strengthens immunity by increasing blood circulation throughout the body. Drinking grape juice on a regular basis will help you lose weight because grapefruit contains high concentrations of vitamin C that act as an antioxidant to release fat stores in your body. Moreover, it also fights malnutrition (malabsorption syndromes like cystic fibrosis, coeliac disease, etc.) and improves overall health by increasing blood circulation in all parts of your body.

Red grapes and red grape juice also contain resveratrol that is loaded with health benefits, especially its antioxidant properties. The compound can help in lowering blood pressure, slow down the age-related cognitive decline, reduce diabetic complications by increasing insulin sensitivity and much more. In fact, the compound has also shown the ability to extend lifespan in animals and might also do the same for humans.

Along with red grape juice, resveratrol is also found in pomegranate and it teams up with bodily tissues to protect the cells against aging. It works wonders for the skin and helps in reducing redness and puffiness too. Resveratrol is undoubtedly your skin's BFF!

9. Pumpkin Juice

Pumpkin is one of the healthy drinks that provide nourishment to an individual by flushing out all the harmful toxins from your body and providing antioxidants. It acts as a powerful detoxifier and helps in improving metabolism, which aids in weight loss. Moreover, it also provides relief from conditions like constipation, colitis, piles, etc., and strengthens immunity by increasing blood circulation throughout the body.

Pumpkin juice can add longevity to your life in many ways. First, it is an excellent source of vitamin A and C, carotenes, etc., which prevent you from chronic diseases like cancer and cardiovascular diseases.

10. Orange Juice

Oranges are known for their refreshing taste and high nutritional benefits due to their unique composition of nutrients like vitamins A & C, lycopene, pectin fiber (a soluble dietary fiber that has been shown to promote healthy digestion), etc. In addition, drinking orange juice on a regular basis will help you lose weight because oranges contain high concentrations of vitamin C that act as an antioxidant to release fat stores in your body. Moreover, oranges fight malnutrition (malabsorption syndromes like cystic fibrosis, coeliac disease) and improve overall health by increasing blood circulation in all parts of your body.

Drinks to avoid for a healthy life:

1. Coffee: Drinking a cup of coffee a day can lead to insomnia, palpitation, and an upset stomach. It also leads to the release of stress hormones that help in fat storage and retention. Moreover, it contains caffeine which is very harmful to pregnant women as they harm their fetus by causing congenital disorders such as cardiac malformations, neural tube defects, etc.

2. Alcohol: Drinking alcohol three times a week decreases your lifespan by up to four years! Apart from this, it also causes liver damage, worsens diabetes mellitus, and increases the risk of developing cancer. Consumption of alcoholic drinks is injurious to health and life-threatening due to its harmful effects on the liver, kidney, pancreas, digestive system, and brain development in children and teenagers. It has been found that alcohol causes life-threatening diseases like cancer, heart attack, digestive disorders, and neurological problems.

3. Sugar-Sweetened Beverages (Soft Drinks): They contain caffeine, artificial sweeteners like aspartame and saccharin that are hazardous for health. These drinks provide zilch nourishment to your body; instead, they act as appetite stimulants by affecting the central nervous system leading to weight gain.

Drinking sugar-sweetened beverages on a regular basis can increase the risk of developing Type II Diabetes by up to 85%, along with obesity, heart disease, and even cancer. This is because it contains high amounts of fructose corn syrup that has harmful effects on your body; it causes insulin resistance which results in fat storage around your waistline, leading to metabolic syndrome and other health issues like diabetes, hypertension, etc.

4. Artificial sweeteners: Artificial sweeteners are toxic to the human body as they contain chemicals like Aspartame (Equal) or Sucralose (Splenda). They affect neurological function by increasing brain tumor risks and also increase the risk of infertility in women by disrupting their reproductive hormones.

5. Energy drinks: Energy drinks are loaded with caffeine which increases stress hormone levels and damages your heart and nervous system over some time. It also leads to mood swings, insomnia, headache, etc.

6. Coffee substitutes: These are caffeinated beverages made from roasted barley or chicory root extract and other ingredients like sugar, caramel color, etc. They contain high amounts of caffeine that can rapidly raise blood pressure levels to weight gain and obesity.

7. Soft drinks: Drinking soft drinks on a regular basis can lead to weight gain by increasing fat storage in the liver, an increased risk of Type II Diabetes, obesity, osteoporosis, and tooth decay. It contains high fructose corn syrup that increases your triglyceride levels leading to insulin resistance which is very harmful to health.

8. Artificial fruit juice: Consuming artificial fruit juices results in added calories with no nutritional benefits because they are made from acidic chemicals like Ascorbic Acid (Vitamin C) or Citric Acid, which contain unhealthy sulfites that cause diarrhea when consumed excessively.

9. Sports Drinks: These beverages are designed to hydrate people who indulge in intense workouts but contain high amounts of electrolytes, which are harmful to health. Apart from that, they also contain sugar, leading to insulin resistance and diabetes.

10. Tea: Drinking tea has its own benefits, but it can have negative effects on your body if consumed excessively because of caffeine content in them which disrupts nervous system activity resulting in insomnia, headache, etc. It also contains tannins that increase cancer risk by disrupting the blood supply to organs and tissues. Moreover, it has a high amount of fluoride, which is toxic for bones leading to skeletal fluorosis.

11. Power drinks: They contain high amounts of electrolytes but lack essential minerals like calcium, magnesium, etc., so they cannot be used for hydration purposes. Moreover, they also contain caffeine that is very harmful to health, as discussed above.

12. Alcoholic beverages: Drinking alcohol on a regular basis can lead to hypertension, stroke, heart disease because it contains toxic chemical ethanol that is made from the distillation of organic materials like potatoes, grains, etc., Moreover, it has high calories that result in an increase in weight, leading to obesity.

13. Diet drinks: People who compulsively drink diet drinks are subjected to addiction. The body adjusts itself only to the taste of artificial sweeteners. It fails to recognize natural sugar consumed, further resulting in drowsiness or sleeplessness, which forces one to consume more caffeine-laden diet drinks. They disrupt your nervous system by interfering with neurotransmitters, resulting in mood swings, anxiety attacks, etc. They also have carcinogenic chemicals in nature which increase the risk of cancer.

With so many options available, sometimes it becomes difficult to decide which of the drinks and beverages are good for health. However, it is essential to include healthy drinks in our daily lives to add longevity and improve health.

Since drinks are one of the major contributors to the longevity of people in the Blue Zone (people who statistically live the longest life without any chronic disease), it is time for you to include them in your daily routine. The second secret of longevity surely works like a charm!

Chapter 3: Healthy Herbs for a Happy Life

Whenever we talk about secrets to a healthy life, we usually come across the importance of healthy fruits, vegetables, and drinks. But, while they add a lot of benefits to our overall health and wellbeing, there is one more secret ingredient that does the same magic- herbs. In Genesis 1:29-30 God said, "I give you every seed-bearing plant on the face of the whole earth and every tree that has fruit with seed in it. They will be yours for food. And to all the beasts of the earth and all the birds in the sky and all the creatures that move along the ground—everything that has the breath of life in it—I give every green plant for food. And it was so. " God provided sustenance for all living creatures in the form of vegetables and herbs. It is we who have long forgotten this truth, and it is time to utilize its benefits.

Botanically, herbs are the leafy parts of plants-fresh or dried used in cooking. Culinary herbs have been used for thousands of years to add flavor to meals while also being used as medicines or preservatives.

Herbs can be used to heal and preserve our bodies as well. Spices like ginger, garlic, and basil are all essential in the culinary world, but they also have their medicinal value.

The health benefits offered by herbs are aplenty, and that's what makes them an important addition to our daily life. This chapter will learn about the plethora of benefits provided by herbs and ways of integrating them into our lives. Let's go!

Top 13 Health benefits of herbs:

1. Treats common cold and fever: Ginger, one of the best herbs, has medicinal properties which help fight against common cold and fever. In addition, the anti-inflammatory properties present in it helps to relieve you from any kind of pain that you might be experiencing due to a cold or fever. To flush the cold virus from your body, drink one cup of boiled mint tea to which you add one shot of vodka and one teaspoon of honey. Chug it and wrap yourself in a blanket from head to toe. You will sweat profusely and the next morning your cold will be gone.

2. Aids digestion: Basil leaves are well known for aiding digestion. They help in the proper functioning of the digestive system and prevent any kind of stomach-related diseases.

3. Gives relief from menstrual cramps: If you are facing problems such as menstrual cramps, then mint can be of great use. The mint's analgesic properties help relieve the pain associated with monthly periods and bring down the inflammation caused due to it.

4. Helps fight cancer: The rich antioxidants present in rosemary helps in preventing cancer. It is very useful in treating leukemia and ovarian cancer.

5. Cleanses the blood: The high amount of vitamin C present in lemongrass acts as a cleanser for our blood by eliminating any toxins accumulated in the body due to environmental pollution or any consumption of non-vegetarian food.

6. Treats tuberculosis: Ginger helps prevent tuberculosis by destroying the bacteria responsible for causing it.

7. Improves digestion: Fennel seeds contain high amounts of dietary fiber along with vitamins A, B, and C, which will enhance digestion by stimulating the production of digestive juices in the stomach.

8. Treats Asthma: Fennel seeds are well known for preventing asthma by getting rid of the phlegm accumulated in the respiratory tracts. Elderberry has been used for centuries around the world to treat asthma. The antiviral properties of this herb help the body fight against any viral infection that might have triggered asthma.

9. Remedy for wounds: Basil leaves help speed up wound healing by destroying harmful bacteria and viruses, which can cause infections at wound sites.

10. Best to aid digestion: Oregano, thyme, and marjoram inhibit the growth of harmful bacteria and promote the growth of good bacteria, which helps in healthy digestion.

11. Treats fungal infections: Tea tree oil is very useful in treating various fungal infections that might affect our skin or body, like athletes' feet, etc.

12. Helps in weight loss: When taken along with meals, Peppermint tea helps promote healthy digestion and boosts your metabolism to aid weight loss.

13. Helps in Vitiligo: Aloe vera is useful as it prevents the occurrence of vitiligo by stimulating the growth of melanin cells, which helps make the skin pigmentation even   again.

Best Herbs to be included in your daily life:

To lead a healthy and long life, we must include these herbs in our daily life:

1. Mint: Herbal tea made out of mint leaves is the best way to reap its benefits. Mint leaves can also be used as a garnish for smoothies. You can also reap its benefits by adding it to your meals while cooking it, which would help stimulate digestive juices in our bodies.

2. Basil: Basil can be used in various ways to get its benefits. It can be included in a curry, salad, or smoothie.

3. Ginger: In order to get the benefits of ginger, you must include it either in your tea or juice. You can also grate some fresh ginger and add it to your salads for added flavor and health benefits.

4. Sage: Sage can be directly consumed in the form of tea or put into your smoothie, salad, or curry to reap its benefits. You can also add ground sage to rice while cooking it. It is best used fresh.

5. Rosemary: Rosemary can be added to your meals in order to get its rich antioxidants. You can also consume it in tea to get rid of any respiratory issues.

6. Lemongrass: Consumption of lemongrass in tea or soup would be beneficial as it rids us from various kinds of infections and skin problems.

7. Oregano: Oregano must be consumed directly through salads, or you can also consume it by adding it to your meals.

8. Thyme: Thyme must be used in the form of soup or tea so that our bodies can reap its benefits. You can also add some thyme while cooking rice for added health benefits

9. Marjoram: Marjoram leaves must be consumed directly in the form of tea or soup. You can also add marjoram while cooking pasta, rice, or vegetables to reap its benefits.

10. Cayenne: Cayenne must be consumed either by adding it to your salads or in the form of herbal tea.

11. Fennel seed: Fennel seeds are best consumed through tea. You can also add fennel seeds to your meals while cooking or salads.

12. Aloe vera: Aloe vera must be consumed directly in the form of juice or through smoothies. It can also be applied to the skin for treating various kinds of wounds, infections, etc.

13. Peppermint: Peppermint oil can be used directly on the skin and is also consumed in the form of tea to treat various kinds of infections and respiratory problems.

14. Chive: Chives are best consumed through salads. They stimulate our digestive juices and help in tackling the problem of blood pressure.

15. Parsley: Parsley can be consumed directly in the form of juice or added to your meals while cooking. It is also used widely as a garnishing herb.

16. Basil: Basil can be consumed directly in the form of juice or as a garnishing herb. You can also add basil to your meals while cooking it. In addition, they help our body by treating a cough and colds.

17. Parsley: The best way to get the benefits of parsley is through juice consumption or in the form of soup. You can also use it as a garnishing herb which would help stimulate digestive juices in our bodies.

18. Cinnamon: When consumed in the form of tea, Cinnamon helps stimulate metabolism and aid weight loss. It also helps in curing a cold and cough.

19. Garlic: Garlic is best consumed in the form of tea. You can also add it to your meals while cooking. Garlic helps our body by preventing heart diseases and various types of cancer. It helps our body by curing problems such as nausea, vomiting, and diarrhea.

Good herb and food combination:

In order to ensure that the benefits of herbs are provided to our body, it is important that they be consumed along with certain foods. For example:

Basil: Basil can be added to any kind of food item while cooking for flavor and attraction. It should, however, be consumed fresh or steeped into a tea. The tea must then be consumed daily. Basil helps in curing respiratory problems and also fights stress. Basil and tomatoes can be blended together to make a sauce that must be added over pasta or any other meal. This would help treat respiratory issues and aid digestion and absorption of essential nutrients.

Sage tea is best consumed after having soup as it helps to improve your digestion and also stimulates the appetite. It treats respiratory issues well too.

Peppermint tea is best paired with food like oatmeal or wheat bread. You can even add peppermint oil to dishes like mashed potatoes, pasta, oatmeal, etc. Peppermint works well in treating respiratory problems and digestive issues.

Oregano is best paired with food like pasta, pizzas, and burgers as it adds a zingy flavor to your food. It also stimulates appetite and treats respiratory issues.

Rosemary can be added to your meals while cooking for better attraction and flavor. In addition, this herb stimulates appetite, treats respiratory problems, and also heals infections.

Thyme can be added to any kind of soup either before or after cooking it. It stimulates appetite, treats respiratory issues, and boosts our body's immune system.

Fennel seed tea is best consumed along with peppermint tea or lemon tea as this combination works well in treating respiratory issues and stimulates appetite. What we eat every day is as important as what we give to our bodies during regular exercises and workouts. Therefore, it is best that we include these healthy herbs in our daily diets for a long and healthy life!

Marjoram: Marjoram is best consumed through tea. It treats respiratory issues and boosts memory power too.

You can consult a professional herbalist to get more information on the right way to use herbs in order to get the maximum benefit from their consumption. You can also buy herbal products online, which would give you access to some of the most powerful herbs.

Lemongrass: Lemongrass helps treat respiratory problems and acts as a natural antidepressant.

You can also get the benefit of lemongrass by adding it to your meals while cooking or garnishing with it. It helps stimulate digestion and appetite too.

Cayenne pepper: Cayenne pepper is best consumed through juice alone. However, if the taste is too strong for you, fruits like oranges can be blended with cayenne pepper to make a juice drink. You can also add it to your meals while cooking them. Cayenne pepper helps stimulate digestion and improves appetite. It also boosts our body's immune system by acting as an anti-inflammatory agent.

Tarragon is best consumed by adding it to food items like pasta, burgers, etc. It helps in curing respiratory problems and also stimulates appetite.

Anise should be added to your meals while cooking them for flavor and attraction. It acts as a powerful antioxidant that detoxifies the body from within. It treats digestive problems well too.

Cloves: Cloves can be steeped into tea or simply consumed raw. This helps treat respiratory problems and also stimulates appetite.

Cinnamon: Cinnamon should be added to your food items while cooking them as it would improve the taste of those particular dishes. It's a known antioxidant that treats digestive issues and boosts immunity too.

Garlic: Garlic is a tasty addition to any meal and is also very healthy for you. It can be used in many ways in your cooking. You can add minced garlic to your sauces, pasta dishes, rice, or vegetables. You can also roast garlic cloves and add them to breads or spreads. If you want a quick and easy way to get the health benefits of garlic, you can simply eat a clove of raw garlic. Be sure to have something to drink with it though, as garlic can be quite potent!

Magic of herbal tea:

Herbal tea is tea made from using any part of a plant for culinary or medicinal purposes. It does not include plain leaves like black, green, etc., which are normally consumed as they are. While loose herbal tea can be directly brewed in water, herbal teas in the form of tea bags are also widely available in markets. Herbal teas taste delicious, are healthy, and can be consumed by people of all ages for treating various kinds of health problems. Many herbs can be used to make herbal tea, for instance, chamomile, peppermint, saffron, etc.

Different companies may offer different types of herbal teas depending upon the region and culture. Herbal teas are also used for various health benefits such as treating respiratory problems, improving digestion skin conditions, and boosting the immune system. Therefore, it is not necessary that one should drink plain water all the time after having a refreshing herbal tea. A healthy combination of herbal tea and food is the best way to improve your immunity and also ensure that you live a long and healthy life.

Tips for cooking with herbs:

Herbs are delicious, fragrant, and flavorful. But when cooked properly with the right ingredients, they can add a whole different aroma and deliciousness to the dish. Here are some of the most common yet powerful tips for cooking with herbs:

1. Dried herbs taste better and are more flavorful than fresh herbs. In general, one teaspoon of dried herbs is equivalent to four teaspoons of fresh herbs.

2. Make small batches of mixed herbs by chopping off the branches and wrapping them in a muslin cloth. While cooking for flavor, you can add these bags and remove them before serving.

3. If you add herbs to rice, make sure that they are boiled first in some water. This would release the flavor of the herb well before adding it to your food.

4. Herbs should be added after the dish has been cooked so as not to lessen its taste or destroy any nutrients.

5. Some herbs are harder in nature than others, such as Cinnamon and rosemary. You should add these herbs at the beginning of the cooking process, and they will retain their flavor throughout the process.

6. Dried whole herbs that are still attached to their stalk are usually more flavorful than loose herbs sold in jars or packets.

7. If you do not want your food to taste garlicky or oniony at all, then you should either steam them before using or fry them first in some oil before putting them into a dish containing food.

8. Herbs such as cilantro and ginger should be used in small quantities when added to dishes. This is because they are very powerful, highly flavored, and aromatic in nature. They can easily alter or destroy the flavors of a dish if overused.

9. If you are cooking with herbs, remember that you must treat them not just like seasoning or garnishing but like fresh ingredients that can alter your dish's taste and flavor.

10. Herbs should be properly dried before storing them for a longer time period. This will prevent them from getting   spoiled earlier   than   their   expected   expiration   date.

Herbs can be used in multiple ways. In all these ways, they add a lot of flavor to every meal while making them healthy for consumption. So make herbs a part of your daily life and enjoy the   healthy   benefits   that   they   have   to   offer.

Chapter 4: Bonding with family- the secret to a long and happy life

The human being is a social animal, and he needs the company of people to be with. The family offers this company. It is the family which gives us support in our times of need .

"This idea of feeling connected becomes very reinforcing, to all of us, and it contributes to happiness, it contributes to mental health and it does contribute also to physical health," says John Northman, a psychologist from Buffalo, NY.

"It's well known that when people feel better connected, that they feel better physically, they're certainly less likely to feel depressed — or if they do, they're in a better position to get out of being depressed. Overall, it leads to a feeling of a greater degree of support and connection psychologically," he said.

A study in the New England Journal of Medicine had shown that stressful family life reduced the lifespan by four months for women and two months for men.

Many examples in our society show how bonding with family adds longevity to our life. Through this chapter, we will understand in detail the importance of positive family time in living a long and healthy life.

Why are families important for individuals?

Family is the best company for human beings. Whether it's love, care, or any other assistance, your family is always there for you. They will support you for various reasons, most of which are likely to be related to your personal wellbeing. Having a healthy relationship with family members such as your spouse and children positively impacts a person's physical, mental, and emotional state. Such support is seldom found anywhere else!

Importance of family for health:

The love and support of your family is a powerful stress reliever. In addition, your affection towards your family works as motivation for fighting diseases or even achieving success in various tasks.

By being with your family, you get to spend your spare time doing something that improves your social life, reduces stress, and keeps you fit.

Along with their regular checkups, your family members play an important role in ensuring your overall health. Thus, even if you are not aware of the changes occurring within your body, it is highly likely that your close ones will guide you towards any suspicious symptoms or diseases.

You can share your secrets only with the ones whom you are close to. You automatically begin to open up and reveal more about yourself when you trust someone. This creates a strong bond between both of you and helps in sharing your issues as well as taking good care of that person if he is unwell. And there is nobody better than the immediate family to develop such strong bonds with!

Being social strengthens immunity- that's why being with family is beneficial. In addition, Socializing reduces stress levels which, in turn, boost immunity to fight diseases.

Your family has the power to change your life for the better by motivating you for a better living! Spending time with your family boosts emotional wellbeing and promotes strong bonds among everyone involved. By being with your family members, you will be able to discuss and resolve any differences with ease. This reduces your stress levels and helps in maintaining a healthy   lifestyle.

Importance of family for mental stability:

Your family will play an important role in maintaining your mental status. Simply spending time with them will make you more relaxed and confident about life. In addition, discussing issues regarding the household with your family helps you to manage all problems easily, thus resulting in peace of mind.

It is true that close interactions with your family members help you overcome any negative thoughts and depression, which in turn reduces the risk of developing stress-related diseases.

A positive atmosphere at home will help you face any challenging situation more confidently! The love, care, and affection that your family displays for you will motivate you to give your best throughout life. And it's fairly easy to keep a strong bond with a supportive family.

Families play an important role in keeping us healthy and happy. Therefore, spending good and quality time with your family will not only strengthen the bond between you and them but also prove to be highly advantageous for your health. Thus, it's not just another day; instead, it ought to be a great opportunity for strengthening your emotional bonds!

Importance of family as a guiding force in life:

In order to achieve goals in life, you need a lot of motivation and support from your family.

Your family acts as a guiding force by providing appropriate solutions for any problem faced by you. Thus, if you are facing problems regarding your career or health, it is advisable to discuss your concerns with your family members as they would be the first ones to know about any changes occurring within your body as well as mind due to their close association; with you since birth!

A supportive family will always motivate and cheer for you, no matter how difficult the situation is. So if you want to succeed in life and face any problem with positivity, try bonding more closely with your family!

Importance of family for spirituality:

Coming together as a family, sharing your happiness and sorrows with each other, praying to god for the wellbeing of everyone present. This way, you can strengthen your bond with your family physically or emotionally and spiritually. This is because spirituality deals with setting up strong emotional connections between people by means of prayer, meditation, or any ritual that could help bind people together in a strong emotional bond!

It brings family members much closer to each other and allows them to share their views regarding god. In turn, this creates a sense of harmony within the four walls of your house, thus encouraging better relationships between family members.

In fact, when you are spiritually connected to your family members, you feel a sense of closeness while being in their company. This creates a positive atmosphere around your house and increases the joy quotient for everyone living under the same roof!

Importance of family for reducing stress:

Spending time with your family is one of the best ways to reduce stress. Even if you meet after a long time, you will be able to share all your thoughts and feelings without any inhibitions. Moreover, this provides an opportunity for everyone present over there to unearth their hidden emotions regarding each other!

A happy and emotionally strong family can bring balance to your life, thus reducing your stress tremendously.

Thus, if you want to get rid of stress and feel better each day, spend more time with the family!

Family closeness helps people live longer:

According to a study, people who have strong ties with their families are likely to live much longer. This is because your family will always be there to support you in every possible way! They will motivate you and encourage you to overcome the problems that life throws at you.

In a long-term study, researchers discovered that many strong family ties were more beneficial than a few strong family relationships, and family ties extended life longer than friendship bonds. It appears that there is something especially unique about family members that provide individuals with the sense of being supported and joyful no one else can.

The most important factor is that it gives you a feeling of belongingness, thereby never letting you feel lonely. So if someone tells you to have close relations with your family for living longer, don't just listen to him/her- rather, follow this mantra religiously!

Impact of our social life on our health

When we think of healthy habits, the first thing that comes to our mind is eating healthy fruits and vegetables, walking those 10,000 steps every day, or hitting the gym regularly. While these are good aspects to maintaining a healthy life, it is equally important to have a good social life that can positively influence our thoughts and overall well being.

Recent research by science writer Marta Zaraska revealed that people with healthy and supportive relationships tend to live longer. In fact, in her studies that spanned an average time period of 7 years, Zaraska found that research participants with a healthy social network were 45% more likely to live longer than the others.

Our mental state has an immediate impact on our bodily functions. Our bodies go through a series of changes when we are stressed, including an increase in cortisol (often known as the "stress hormone") and the activation of our cardiovascular system's "fight or flight" response.

Loneliness is one of the most significant stressors that humans face, and it has an impact on our biological systems. For example, cortisol and inflammation have been found to increase due to loneliness, which is detrimental to our health over time. Participants were exposed to a cold virus in one research, and researchers tracked their symptoms. The result?

People who were socially isolated in life had a 45 percent increased chance of getting sick.

Taking time to connect with others may help trigger better biological processes, such as the release of oxytocin, in response to stress and loneliness. Oxytocin has been linked to a variety of benefits, including lowering cortisol and pain, altering how our brains react to potential stressors, and even stimulating the growth of new brain cells.

Because our social connections are so essential for our health, it's critical to devote time to thinking about how to enhance them. It's probably no surprise that learning and practicing gratitude have been shown to improve your mental health. But did you know that doing so might also boost your physical health? Kindness is just as important for your mind, body, and spirit as it is for other aspects of life (such as meal-planning or training for a 5K), so there's no doubt that maintaining a positive and healthy community around you is important for your good health.

Other benefits of having a good social life

There are numerous other benefits of having a healthy social life. Let us take a look at some of them:

1. Being social helps us as we age:

Having low stress and a healthy social life can help us years after retiring. Many researchers argue that it is possible to fall into the trap of becoming isolated during retirement and face "empty nest syndrome," where there is no one left at home, and we lose our sense of purpose in life. A study conducted with retirees at 62 found that those with low social connections had a higher mortality rate than those who were more socially engaged.

In fact, a study published in Psychology and Aging revealed that social butterflies are generally happier with their lives during their golden years.

2. Being social may help in staving off diseases:

Studies suggest that having a social life can help prevent us from developing high blood pressure in the future. For example, a study published by the University of Minnesota Medical School revealed that having a healthy social life can decrease the risk of cardiovascular disease, reduce stress and boost recovery after heart surgery.

Another research suggests that those with close relationships may even have stronger immune systems to fight off infections as well as live healthier lives. In fact, people who were living alone had a 10 to 30 percent, and those who lived with a spouse had a 3-6 percent increased risk of illness than those who lived with others.

All these facts clearly point out how important it is to have a healthy social life in order to boost your overall well being.

3. Being social can help us live happier:

A University of Michigan longitudinal study of 1,000 people found that those who had strong social lives were more likely to report "high levels of happiness and life satisfaction" than those who didn't. Another study published in the Journal of Socio-Economics revealed that we tend to enjoy life more when we're surrounded by our friends, family, and acquaintances.

The bottom line is that relationships are absolutely essential for good mental health. Whether it's your spouse, your children, or even your neighbors, you need to have a strong social support system if you want to live a happy and healthy life.

4. Socializing is great for our mental health too.

Having a good social life has been associated with better moods over time, better results at work, and enhanced cognitive functions. For example, a 2001 study found that married people experience less anger, stress, and depression than those who live alone. And a 2004 study revealed that people with strong social networks have enhanced mental abilities and perform better at work.

In short, being socially active is good for both our mental health as well as longevity.

So what are you waiting for? First, get off your couch and join a club or start an activity that you usually love doing. Then, engage in these activities with your friends and family and foster your social relationships and family bonding for greater fun. That way, you will be able to reap the benefits of having a healthy social life, and we can all enjoy a long and happy life.

Chapter 5: Golden sleep for a longer life

Sleep is a very busy time for your body. It might sound counterintuitive, but it is the time when many important processes are at work that support everything from our cardiovascular system to our neural functions. Sleep on the floor on a Japanese style mattress not more than 1 inch thick.

Though the sleep needs vary from person to person, adults usually require an undisturbed sleep of 7-9 hours every day. The optimum regimen is to sleep at the same time everyday and to retire with the sun and rise with the sun. However, most people are deprived of this amount due to factors like work pressure, stress, pollution, and irregular eating habits.

The lack of sound sleep can have adverse effects on your physical as well as mental health. In addition, it may lead to several chronic diseases, including obesity, diabetes, depression, etc., which are harmful to your overall longevity.

In this chapter, we will learn about the importance of sleep on our health and longevity while also discovering ways to improve the quality of sleep. Let's go!

Why does your body need sleep?

Sleep aims not merely to make you feel more refreshed but also to allow your muscles, organs, and brain cells to repair and rejuvenate every night. In addition, sleep helps control your metabolism and regulate the hormones that are released from your body. When these processes are disturbed by lack of sleep, it raises the danger of disease.

Sleeping for less than seven hours per night puts you at risk of being involved in deadly accidents. According to 2014 research, sleeping six hours each night raises the likelihood of having a vehicle accident by 33 percent compared to sleeping seven or eight hours each night. The researchers determined that 9% of all motor vehicle incidents may be linked to people who sleep fewer than seven hours per night.

When you sleep, the body and your brain enter a restorative cycle. During this time, your muscles and bones are strong and restore themselves, while toxins are removed from the body through breathing and other bodily functions. Proper sleep also helps in the better digestion of food which is vital for maintaining good health.

The Hidden Cost of insufficient sleep

When individuals are pressed for time, sleep is frequently one of the first things to suffer. Many people regard sleep as a luxury and believe that the benefits of restricting their sleeping hours outweigh the drawbacks. People frequently overlook the long-term health consequences of insufficient sleep and how poor health can impact one's productivity over time.

Poor sleep has a variety of hidden costs. Obesity, diabetes, and cardiovascular disease are all linked to medical issues that develop over time and are caused by a number of variables, including genetics, poor diet, and inactivity. Insufficient sleep has also been linked to a variety of illnesses, and it is viewed as a significant risk factor. Getting enough restful sleep may be as crucial to one's health and well-being as eating properly and exercising.

Risks associated with lack of proper sleep:

Improper sleep exposes us to various health problems, and scientific research has concluded them many times. Here is a roundup of the most common risks associated with the lack of proper sleep:

1. Obesity: Sleeping less than 7 hours a night can significantly impact your weight. It increases the hormone cortisol, which triggers fat storage around the waistline and elevates sugar levels in the blood. Sufficient sleep is linked to weight gain in a variety of ways. One study discovered that individuals who slept fewer than six hours on a regular basis were considerably more likely to have excess body fat. In contrast, those who slept nine or more hours had the lowest proportion of relative body fat among the study group. Another research revealed that babies who are considered "short sleepers" are far more likely to become overweight as young adults than those who sleep for the recommended amount.

2. Diabetes: Sleep deprivation makes you more prone to the risk of diabetes. The researchers found that people who slept for about 6 hours each night were 23 percent more likely to develop Type 2 diabetes than those who got 7-8 hours of sleep. Fortunately, improved sleep has also been linked to better blood sugar control and the prevention of type 2 diabetes.

3. Depression: Insufficient sleep can elevate your risks of depression by almost 50%, according to research done on students. The study involved questionnaires from more than 4,000 students about their sleeping patterns and symptoms of depression. They found that those who slept for five hours or less every night were 47% more likely to develop symptoms of depression. According to another research, people with insomnia are at a greater risk of developing clinical depression over time.

4. Cardiovascular diseases and hypertension: According to recent research, 6 to 7 hours of sleep per night was linked to a 2.4-times higher risk of coronary artery calcification, which is a predictor of future myocardial infarction (heart attack) and death from heart disease. Obstructive sleep apnea has also been linked to an increased risk of cardiovascular diseases, including hypertension, stroke, coronary heart disease, and arrhythmia.

5. Immune function: Researchers have found that sleep deprivation hinders the immune system. A study published in Annals of Internal Medicine concluded that being awake for more than 19 hours impairs one's immune function as severely as being under the influence of alcohol.

Health risks of too much sleep

It's not just a lack of sleep that has negative consequences. Sleeping too much might also be indicative of health issues. In one research, sleeping for a long period—defined as more than 10 hours each night—was linked to psychiatric illnesses and being overweight, but it was not associated with other chronic medical problems related to insufficient sleep.

According to one research, sleeping nine or more hours a night was linked to a 23% higher chance of stroke. In addition, those who slept for more than 9 hours and napped for at least 90 minutes during the day had an 85 percent increased risk of stroke.

It might be an indication that something is wrong if you constantly require more sleep. Excess drowsiness might be the consequence of numerous factors, including sleep disorders and sleep apnea, which can all cause an insufficient overall quality of rest. To evaluate your sleeping habits, you should see a medical expert in this instance.

Excessive sleeping (or not enough sleep, or with early-morning awakenings) might also be a symptom of depression. However, occasionally more apparent manifestations of sadness are not evident; it is crucial to discuss this with a medical professional.

Best sleep duration for longevity

According to studies, the optimum amount of sleep per night is seven to eight hours. However, each person's required amount of sleep varies. Genetics, personality, stress, and other factors may play a role in determining how much sleep people need. Some lucky ones can function on five or six hours of rest each night, while others might require nine or ten hours of sleep every night to feel happy and healthy.

Recommending the same amount of slumber for everyone is difficult because it varies from person to person. However, the National Sleep Foundation suggests that you should go to bed at a time when you usually become tired and get up at a time which leaves you refreshed in the morning.

However, we must complete a sleep cycle of at least 7 hours in order to carry out the daily chores properly without compromising our health.

The relationship between sleep and age

It is not surprising that the older people get, the more likely they are to report various sleep problems. Some of these complaints can even be a sign of an undiagnosed health problem like Alzheimer's disease or dementia.

What you should remember about your sleep as you age:

When we grow old, we tend to sleep less and typically take longer to fall asleep for two reasons:

•As we get older, the amount of time spent in deep slow-wave sleep decreases.

•Older people often experience less restful sleep than younger people due to a limited ability to consolidate their stages of sleep.

Adults between the ages of 18 and 64 need 7 to 9 hours of sleep each night.

Even though teens may not be able to fall asleep when they want, they should get 8-10 hours of sleep every day in order for their brains and bodies to function properly.

Top 10 benefits of a sound sleep

Sleep deprivation can put your health and safety in danger, which is why it's critical to prioritize and protect your sleep on a daily basis. This part goes into ten reasons why you should get more sleep.

1. Can help you in maintaining or losing weight:

Getting enough sleep can contribute to a healthy weight and decrease the risk of obesity, heart disease, and diabetes over time. One main reason: When we get less than 7 hours of sleep per night, our levels of ghrelin (the "hunger hormone") increase; this makes it more likely that we will overeat.

Sleep deprivation has been linked to increased weight gain, and it is influenced by a variety of variables, including hormones and motivation to exercise. Sleep deprivation, for example, increases ghrelin levels and reduces leptin levels. Ghrelin is a hormone that makes us feel hungry, while leptin is a hormone that makes us feel full. This may cause us to feel hungrier and overeat as a result of rising hunger hormones such as ghrelin and declining appetite suppressants like leptin.

This is backed by numerous research, which reveals that sleep-deprived individuals have a greater appetite and eat more calories. Furthermore, sleep deprivation causes you to desire higher in sugar and fat meals due to their greater calorie content.

Worse yet, if you had a night of insufficient sleep, you may be less inclined to go to the gym, walk outdoors, or execute whatever other physical effort you enjoy.

As a result, prioritizing sleep may assist in the maintenance of healthy body weight.

2. Can improve the concentration and productivity levels:

    The negative effects of sleep deprivation can propagate into your work or school performance. For example, research has found that sleep-deprived students show poor grades in school and have lower standardized test scores than their well-rested peers.

    As you might imagine, if your cognitive functions are impaired by not getting sufficient hours of sleep, you'll have a tough time concentrating and helping to advance your career or education.

    Finally, children and adults who have adequate sleep have been shown to do better in problem-solving and memory tasks.

3. Can help in maximizing your athletic performance:

    Sleep-deprived people typically experience a decline in their physical performance, including anaerobic activities such as sprinting and weightlifting. On the other hand, athletes whose training schedules prioritize sufficient hours of slumber have been shown to have better reaction times on the playing field.

Numerous studies have shown Adequate sleep to improve fine motor abilities, reaction time, muscular power, muscular endurance, and problem-solving skills. Furthermore, lack of sleep might increase your risk of injury and reduce your desire to exercise.

As you learned in the sections above, sleep deprivation can reduce your performance. So, if you're having trouble performing at your best due to lack of sleep, consider taking a closer look at your schedule to see whether anything could be done about it.

4. Can help in strengthening your heart:

   Sound sleep also plays a significant role in protecting your heart. In fact, research has found that people who don't get enough sleep are at increased risk of high blood pressure and cardiovascular disease. Moreover, when you're deprived of sleep, your body releases higher levels of stress hormones such as cortisol and adrenaline, even if you're not in danger.

   In subsequent research, researchers have found that stress hormones could make blood pressure rise or fall erratically. In addition, elevated stress hormones could boost the level of triglycerides in your bloodstream, increasing your risk of heart disease. Furthermore, sleep deprivation can lead to endothelial dysfunction by decreasing nitric oxide production and increasing oxidative stress—two processes that can lead to atherosclerosis.

Endothelial dysfunction is a disease process in which the inner lining of your arteries, called the endothelium, becomes damaged and less efficient for transporting nutrients and waste products throughout your body.

So, sleep for 8 hours every day to keep your body fit and heart   healthy.

5. Can reduce instances of inflammation:

When you're sleep-deprived, your body's inflammatory response system becomes activated more than it should. As a result, the immune cells in your body start to release high levels of pro-inflammatory cytokines and molecules that can actually disrupt normal blood flow. All of this is believed to play a significant role in the development of certain chronic diseases.

Additionally, sleep deprivation can worsen existing inflammatory conditions such as asthma, rheumatoid arthritis, psoriasis, irritable bowel syndrome, and even gum disease. On the other hand, people who regularly get a good night's rest can lower their diabetes and heart disease risk.

Sleeping well helps to combat chronic disease.

6. Can positively impact emotions and social interactions:

   Few people realize that sleep deprivation can profoundly impact your emotional state. For instance, lack of sleep can boost the levels of stress hormones in your body while decreasing feel-good neurotransmitters such as serotonin, leading to moodiness and irritability.

   In fact, research has found that inadequate slumber could worsen depression symptoms. It could also lead to increased anxiety and hostility.

   Sleeping well not only helps you feel better, but it could also help improve your relationships with family and friends.

Quick tips to sleep better at night

If you aren't currently getting the sleep you need, here are some tips for you to enjoy a healthy and sound sleep:

1. Start with creating a sleep-friendly environment:

   Create an environment that's ideal for restful sleep. For instance, studies show that exposure to light at night can adversely affect circadian rhythms and suppress the production of melatonin—a hormone that regulates your body's internal clock. So, it is recommended to turn off all the electronic gadgets before heading towards the bed as they emit blue light that could interfere with sleep quality. In addition, consuming alcohol or caffeine can also interfere with your sleep as well as cause other complications.

2. Sleeping in a dark room can help you get better and sound sleep:

    It's important to make your bedroom conducive for sleep. If possible, eliminate distractions such as noise and light pollution in the bedroom. Keep the room dark, quiet, and cool (at or below 65 degrees Fahrenheit). Also, remove any TVs or other gadgets that emit blue light from your bedroom.

3. Establishing a regular sleeping routine:

    A regular sleeping routine is equally important to ensure an uninterrupted and refreshing sleep. To be precise, having a consistent bedtime schedule can improve your overall quality of sleep. You should stick to the same hours every night and day to your body's internal rhythms—the so-called circadian rhythms.

4. Avoid heavy meals before bedtime:

    Besides this, if you are trying to lose weight or simply want to get better sleep at night, it is important that you avoid heavy meals before bedtime. Instead, your meal should be light and easily digestible as it lets your stomach muscles relax and not strain on breaking down a heavy meal.

5. Sleeping without disturbance is important for good sleep:

Trying to limit the amount of time spent in bed, but make sure you keep your body relaxed during this time. For instance, spending ten hours in bed during the weekend but sleeping for only six to eight hours could make your body accustomed to less sleep every day except on weekends. Eventually, this could lead to insomnia. Also, if you tend to use your laptop, tablet, or phone just before going to bed, it could have a negative effect on your quality of sleep as it can cause disruptions in melatonin production. So, it is necessary that you should spend about 85 percent of your time in bed asleep rather than just lying there.

Chapter 6: Exercise is the key to a healthier life

Do you want to feel good, increase your energy levels, and even add years to your life? The way to do all this is simple: Just exercise!

Any activity that makes your muscles work and demands that you use calories to fuel it is considered exercise. Swimming, running, jogging, walking, and dancing are just a few examples of physical activities. The most important thing to remember about exercise is that any amount is better than none. Even just a few minutes of activity every day helps stave off disease and maintain your health. If you wait until you have more time, though, days or weeks may pass before you get around to exercising again! And the longer you go between workouts, the harder it will be to get back into your exercise routine. Through this chapter, you will understand the importance of exercise in maintaining a healthy life and explore various simple exercises that can be easily integrated into our daily lives.

Why Exercise Matters

Getting and staying physically active is one of the most important lifestyle adjustments you can make to lower your risk of getting many age-related diseases while increasing your chance of remaining active and independent. Physical activity is one of the most significant of these. With daily exercise, it is possible to:

1. Control your weight: Exercise makes the muscles work, which consumes calories. If you are able to maintain muscle mass through exercise, your body will burn more calories at rest, even when you are sleeping. This helps maintain a healthy weight or maybe even reduces your weight because it increases the rate of fat loss.

2. Control high blood pressure: Exercise can help keep it in check if you have high blood pressure. Being active boosts high-density lipoprotein (HDL) cholesterol and lowers harmful triglycerides, no matter your current weight. This one-two punch keeps your blood flowing properly, lowering your risk of heart disease while controlling your blood pressure levels.

3. Prevent bone loss: Bone is constantly changing, with old bone being broken down and new bone is formed. Exercise stimulates the growth of new bone. Without it, bones tend to break down faster than they rebuild themselves. This results in reduced height, osteoporosis (a disease that causes bones to become fragile), or fractures.

4. Increase your chances of living longer: People who are physically active live the longest, with one study showing that activity levels have a greater impact on life

span than whether you smoke, have high cholesterol, or are   overweight.

5. Prevent type 2 diabetes: People who exercise regularly are less likely to develop type 2 diabetes, and those with diabetes can benefit from exercise as well. Exercise helps control blood sugar levels (not only will it keep your levels in a normal range, but it may help you avoid the disease altogether), and insulin sensitivity increases after you exercise. Daily exercise helps to control blood sugar and prevent this disease. Remember that physical activity is not limited to traditional exercise. Any physical activity counts, so you must include some form of   daily   activity   in   your   life.

6. Boosts energy: Having more energy and feeling better is an added bonus of regular activity. Exercise can also help you sleep better at night, so it provides a double benefit by increasing the quality of your rest as well.

7. Keeps your brain sharp: Exercise has been shown to prevent age-related memory loss and can reverse some of the effects of Alzheimer's disease. Exercising has been found to cause the hippocampus, a brain structure important for memory and learning, to develop in size.

8. Stay active and independent: Exercise improves strength, balance, coordination, and flexibility. With regular exercise, you are more likely to be able to do the things you love to do every day—getting dressed in the morning without difficulty or enjoying a game of catch with your kids at the park.

9. Increase the quality of life: Anyone can see that daily exercise makes you feel better. Regular activity boosts energy, improves mood, helps you get a good night's rest, and gives you more confidence to take on the world.

10. Improve your sleep: Sleep is critical for our well-being. Getting enough sleep can help you maintain a healthy weight, improve your mood and mental health, regulate hormones that control appetite and energy levels, increase your creativity and problem-solving ability. When you exercise daily, it helps you relax and fall asleep faster at night.

11. Increase your fitness level: If you are physically active, you will become more fit, burning off stress and improving your mood in the process. Even if you never lace up your running shoes again once this program is over, the habits of regular physical activity will last for a

lifetime.

How much exercise is enough?

You can choose from many different types of activities: walking, jogging, cycling, swimming, dancing; anything that gets you moving and increases your heart rate is considered exercise. You will want to do whatever you enjoy and can do on a regular basis.

While exercising, breathe through your belly which is called diaphragmatic breathing. This proper breathing starts in the nose and then moves to the stomach as your diaphragm contracts, the belly expands and your lungs fill with air. The diaphragm pulls down on the lungs, creating negative pressure in the chest, resulting in air flowing into your lungs. Watch a baby breathe. The baby naturally uses the diaphragm to breathe. Focus on a spot two inches below your belly-button and inhale from that point. That's how a baby breathes without even thinking about it.

You don't need to set aside long blocks of time; even short bursts of activity throughout the day will make a big difference in your health and energy level.

Three components: The activities that you do every day—like climbing stairs, cooking dinner, or walking from your car to the mall—are considered daily physical activity (DPA).

Aerobic exercise: Aerobic activities get your heart pumping and increase the flow of oxygen to all parts of your body. Running, cycling, swimming, or dancing are examples of aerobic exercises. You'll notice an improvement in your overall health and fitness if you include some aerobic activity in your life.

Also, **resistance training**: Muscle strength and endurance improve with weight training—or what some people call "strength training" or "resistance exercise." Strength-training activities that you may want to consider include the use of weights, machines at a health club, elastic bands, bodyweight exercises such as pushups, or activities such as rock climbing which uses your own body weight for resistance.

Strength training: Strength-training activities are done with free weights or resistance machines. You can use hand-held weights, weight stacks at a gym, your own body weight (e.g., pushups), elastic bands, or some combination of these types of weights to strengthen your muscles during aerobic activity.

Play: Regardless of age, most people think they don't have time to be active, but physical activity doesn't necessarily mean running a marathon or taking an aerobics class. You can get lots of physical activity throughout the day by using your body in everyday life. Try to find ways to move more— take the stairs instead of the elevator, walk instead of driving short distances, clean the house vigorously and carry heavy loads up and downstairs.

Simple exercises to integrate into your daily life:

You don't need to be an exceptional sportsman to extend your life. However, regular, moderate exercises such as fast walking have been linked to several years of longer life. Here are some simple yet effective exercises that you can integrate into your daily life and improve your overall health:

1. Cycling: Cycling is a great way to get around. It places no strain on the back or neck, gives the hamstrings and calf muscles a good workout without any impact at all, can be done by people of almost any age, young children included!

2. Walk upstairs instead of using the lift/elevator: Stair climbing at the rate of 1,500 steps per day can boost

your health by reducing the risk of obesity, high cholesterol, Type-2 diabetes, heart disease, and even cancer.

3. Walk instead of driving: You could improve your heart and lung fitness levels by walking or cycling to work or school as often as you can. If you live too far away from your place of employment or school, try walking there on weekends. Try to walk ten thousand steps per day.

4. Do household chores vigorously: Housework such as scrubbing floors, mopping, and sweeping can be a great form of moderate exercise if you do it vigorously enough. If you don't want to break your back doing heavy housework all at once, then try splitting chores into several five-minute periods throughout the day.

5. Pick up small objects off the floor: An easy way to get fitness is to pick up objects off the floor. Try not to use a dustpan or broom, but bend down with your hands and knees!

6. Do yard work on sunny days: Yard work such as mowing the lawn on sunny days can be an excellent source of moderate exercise. But make sure you don't overdo it by straining yourself or spending too long

doing   it.

7. Stretching: Stretching every day can not only improve your flexibility it can also reduce tension and stress. You don't have to get into complicated positions or maintain any special body postures. Just stretch for 10 minutes in the morning while you're watching television or listening   to   music.

8. Squatting: Squatting is a great way to ease daily aches and pains. Squatting reduces the pressure on your back, decreases tension in the head of your thighbones, stretches calf muscles and Achilles' tendons, gets hip flexors moving again. It also stretches adductor muscles that run along the inside of the thighs, loosens up hips and knees and strengthens the muscles of your buttocks.

9. Take the stairs instead of the elevator: You don't need to become a marathon runner or an athlete to increase your level of fitness. In fact, you should aim to be slightly more active every day to keep fit. One way to do this is by making use of your daily routine. For example, if you use the elevator to move one floor in a building, take the stairs instead of on your way back. Or, if you usually leave work and head straight for the train

station, try walking home instead. This simple change of routine will positively affect your fitness without taking too much time out of your daily schedule.

10. Plank hold: The plank hold is a great way to enhance your balance and stability while also improving core strength. It can be used by anyone looking for a simple, no equipment required exercise.

11. Crunches: Crunches are an effective way of strengthening muscles that support the back and spine. In fact, they're so good that it's recommended that everyone should do them every day to maintain the shape of his or her core.

The bottom line

Regular exercise has several advantages that may enhance almost every aspect of your health. For example, regular exercise can boost the production of hormones that make you feel happier and help you sleep better.

It's also beneficial for:

- improving the appearance of your skin

- helping you in losing or maintaining body weight and BMR

- reducing the risk of cardiovascular and other chronic diseases

- improving your mental health

It only takes a little movement to make a significant difference in your health.

If you want to meet the fitness and activity guidelines set by the Department of Health and Human Services for adults, aim for 150 to 300 minutes of moderate-intensity exercise each week or 75 minutes of vigorous exercise every week.

Moderate-intensity aerobic exercise is any activity that makes your heart beat faster, such as walking, cycling, or swimming. Running and doing a strenuous fitness class are examples of vigorous-intensity activities.

Make sure you include at least two days of muscle-strengthening exercises that work all major muscle groups (legs, hips, back and abdomen, chest, shoulders, and arms), and you'll surpass the guidelines.

Barbells, dumbbells, resistance bands, and your own body weight may all be used to perform muscular strengthening exercises. Squats, pushups, shoulder presses, chest presses, and planks are examples of these.

Regardless of what you do for a living or whether you stick to the idea of 150 minutes of activity per week, you may still improve your health in various ways.

Chapter 7: Mental Health: Foundation for a Long Life

Life maneuvers through the food and habits we consume, and we reap benefits if we are sincere about what we do. But a strong physique, a loving environment, and genuine people around you will become meaningless if you do not have a healthy mind. It is a basement on which you lay upon your whole life. Every shortcoming and hurdle in your life can take a toll on your lifespan.

Your real strength doesn't come from what your body can endure but from how much your mind can endure. You have been there! When all you built inside, your heart went shattering into pieces. Your usual strong persona turned into a fragile glass, and you sat there as vulnerable as a glass toy. So why did it happen? Are you not capable? No. It was not because you are weak, but because you didn't prepare yourself for it.

This seventh rule will help you to strengthen the inner you. There is a spirit capable of sustaining the worst of the worst. All you need is a nudge to awaken it. The world is moving towards technology and comfort. Simultaneously, we are detaching ourselves from Nature. How often do you take the time to listen to Nature? No one is to be blamed. Life just evolved.

In this chapter, we will see a way to connect with your inner soul. I am not proposing a complex solution but simple yet forgotten ways. You aspire! But it doesn't cross the level of being a goal until you put it into practice. Hence, I propose a way to establish such healthy practices that can impart a healthier life.

Meditation to Awaken Yourselves

The start of the day is like the first impression to the rest of the day. As we say, if you are to impress someone, you should be thoughtful during the first meeting. Why is it important?

Let us presume you see a person in ragged clothes snapping at everyone he sees. In reality, he might be a hardworking person who is good at heart, toiling for his family. His foul mood can be because of all his workload and stress from survival. But you wouldn't know it. The moment you see him, you become unimpressive. It is applied to the start of the day as well.

You should weed out all the negativity in your life. It is a new day, and it possesses a lot more opportunities. Hence, there is no point in carrying it over to the rest of the day.

Meditation is a powerful tool with very little recognition that can overwhelm you with all the energy you need to survive the rest of the day. Morning, when you wake up after a good sleep, you will possess maximum energy. The mind will be like a clean slate. Hence, it is the right time to practice mediation. By doing so, you can preserve all the power and peace of mind throughout the day.

Meditation is more than just a practice. It rejuvenates you from the inside out. It is not just a spiritual aspect of life; it has its proven science. It has many advantages like

1. Stress reduction

2. Anxiety reduction

3. Memory retention

4. Increasing self-awareness

5. Betterment of emotional well-being

6. Memory enhancement

7. Boosts-up positivity

8. Overcoming addictions

9. Solving sleep disorders

10. Overcoming pain

11. Maintaining blood pressure

12. Strengthening the thoughts

You have an unexplored ability within you that lays dormant. Mediation can ignite it to utilize the maximum capacity.

So, what is the right time to do meditation? It is the moment you open your eyes!! It is the first thing you should be doing in the morning. The toughest thing is taking the first step. Once you do, you will be there in no time.

If you think you will get the calmness of the mind as soon as you close your eyes, no! You got it all wrong! It is a long process. It takes days or even months to establish such a kind of expertise. There are different ways in which you can do meditation. You can either do it by sitting or lying down. It is the choice you can make at your convenience. The important thing is whatever you choose, you should be able to listen to yourself.

The moment we think about meditation, many of us come to the conclusion that it is something we do to eliminate all thoughts from our minds. In a way, it may be true as we streamline ours through mediation. But you cannot force yourself to throw out all the thoughts completely. As you know, the human mind can be crazy! The more you try to resist, the more desirable it will become. Hence I propose simple techniques which you can follow to establish a meditation routine.

1. Give it a purpose

For every morning, you can have one thing in mind, on which you can try to establish it in your mind. You can try thinking about a red rose, a sunset, or a star-filled sky. You can put your effort into visualizing the thing or mercenary you choose and picture it inside your mind. It is easier than getting rid of the thoughts. Instead, you will be diverting your mind to the thought of your choice.

2. It is ok to move

Meditation doesn't necessarily mean gluing yourself to one place. There are types of mediation that recommend movement and still establish self-awareness.

If you feel sitting at one place or being idle is not your cup of tea, you can choose to move and still meditate. You can imbibe meditation into yoga which is efficient in tackling stress. Apart from it, there are three major types of movement yoga.

1. Walking Meditation

2. Qigong

3. Tai Chi

In all the above three-movement meditation, there will be interaction with the outside world. It involves slower movement than usual while holding the consciousness of mind and body. It enlightens the "chi," as the Chinese call it, which is the internal energy of a soul.

4. Do it along with music or chants.

Do the sounds of the outside world annoys you? Then you can couple your meditation along with the music. There is a variety of music for meditation purposes, and you can make a pick of your taste. You can also use chants of "Om" or "Um" in the form of music or by saying it aloud. The vibrations the chants and the music can create are quite refreshing to the mind and thoughts. It can make you feel all the energy flowing inside your body.

5. Lying down on the floor

Meditation can be done even while lying down if you feel that it is comfortable for you. It is even easy to do when you wake up in the morning. I would recommend doing it on the floor with a yoga mat on. Try lying down on the floor facing up. Make sure to loosen your body and relax it from head to toe, and close your eyes. It is often referred to as "Yoga Nidra." As you close your eyes, concentrate on your mind and body, one at a time. It will ease your whole body and will help you see your body as a third person.

6. Take Aid of the Counts

Not everyone is a self-starter; it will feel like it is better to have a guide. Yes! You can have one. Keep the counting as your guide. If you are confused about how and where to start the meditation, the best thing is by count. It is not essentially mandatory to close your eyes while meditating; you keep it fixed on an object for better concentration.

Start with the count of 1 and move forward with the count for every inhale and exhale. Try to do it as slowly and deeply as possible. Keep the counting cycle to 10, and start from 1 after every 10th count.

Don't keep your concentration on your count, and it is ok to lose your count a little bit. Instead, focus on your body and your breathing, and listen to what your body says. The count will avoid distraction and will keep your practice intact.

7. Listen to Yourself

The ultimate aim of meditation is self-consciousness. Breather your belly, that is , breathe with your diaphragm. Hence whatever method you are using, just be aware of your body. You should pay attention to every part of your body, from head to toe. As you learn to observe your body, you will learn to familiarize your body. It will lead to a connection with your soul and mind. As you practice every day, you will master the control of your body.

8. Keep it Short

Sitting in a place, maintaining a posture, and concentrating is not an easy thing. So move on by taking baby steps. Even if you are able to accomplish it in 5 minutes, it is big. So it is ok to start from as low as 1 minute and grow up the ladder. There is no specific time duration for doing meditation. What is important here is doing it on a consistent basis.

9. Give it time

Loving the process is more important in life than whatever you do. Isn't it? When you drink coffee to feel refreshed and relaxed, you take your time savoring the aroma and taste by sipping it little by little. Meditation should give you the same experience.

You should do it by realizing its importance and letting the effect flow through your body. So do not force yourself at any point of the time, and accept that everything takes time. The first few days, you might find your mind wavering despite your efforts. But it is natural; you will become more focused as your practice every day.

10.   Wim Hof's Way

Wim Hof took the meditation to the next level by imbuing simplicity and science to it. It involves three components that make your meditation and breathing habit more refined and efficient.

1. Breathing - Even though we have been breathing all our life, we are hardly aware of it. Being able to listen to it and streamline it increases the better flow of oxygen in the body.

2. Step 1: Choose the choice of posture, like lying down or sitting, and make yourself at ease.

3. Step 2: Start the inhalation through your mouth or nose and take it as deep as possible through your belly. As you release it, keep it natural and let it out without putting any effort. As you do it, you can feel a new sensation in your body. It can either cause tingles or dizziness, but it is quite natural. Make at least 40 counts of the process.

4. Step 3: After you do it at least 40 times, hold your breath after the exhale. Try to endure it as long as possible and let it go when you can't do it anymore.

5. Step 4: Inhale as much as possible until you get the feel of filling your lungs, hold it as much as for 15 sec and release it. This makes a count of one cycle. Try doing three or four cycles in the uninterrupted cycle.

6. Cold Therapy: Wim Hof emphasizes the importance of coldness in treating the body. Studies have shown the path to fat loss, inflammation reduction, and mood elevation through exposure to cold. Hence he recommends doing the breathing exercise in cold

regions. If you think you cannot do it on the outside ice, you can start with cold showers.

7. Commitment: As the natural rule, every success and benefit arrives with sincerity and consistency. The cold exposure increases one's will and pushes one to go beyond their limits. Stronger is your will, better is your life decisions. You can create a better version of yourself.

Journaling: A secret Room To your Thoughts

The end of the day is usually the most chaotic and emotional time. You will be brimming with thoughts of the whole day, or someday of the whole life. Not every thought in mind is meant to be talked about, but it needs to be let out. Also, there are things you want to remember and be reminded of forever, yet you tend to forget them amidst your busy and pressing schedule. Journaling is a handy friend to tackle your thoughts. Yes, I hear You sigh! Are you making me write a whole long story every day? No. Certainly not!

There are no hard or soft rules to writing a journal; you can just write whatever way it makes you comfortable. It is not always about making detailed comprehension; you can improvise it. You can even write it like it is an Instagram post or Facebook boost. You can even doodle it! But it is important to record your thoughts.

When you write what is agitating and burdening in your mind, you will contemplate your thoughts. It is way better than dealing with it within your mind. Telling it to another person might raise conflicting thoughts. But when you write, you keep it to yourself, yet you tend to find a solution. In the end, your mind will be free from opposing and disturbing thoughts. You will feel your mind light like a feather.

Gratitude Journal

I already said a journal can help you keep calm which in turn leads to a long life. So, why a gratitude journal? More importantly, what is that? It is simple! It is a way to hammer the positive thoughts in your life.

It is the kind of journal you would want to preserve forever. In this journal, you will write only positive things that happened on that day. To be effective, make yourself write at least three things for a day. As you start writing day by day, you might feel like repeating the things already written, but no. You should not do that. You don't need to find anything big to be mentioned in it. It can be as tiny as eating a candy you love.

This process will make you appreciate the good things in your life. It will take you to the realization that there are "n" number of things in your life that make it worth fighting for. As you go on and on, you will start noticing the things happening in your life keenly and become aware of yourself and your surroundings. You can even mention the people who made you smile that day or a dream that made you feel happy.

3-6-9 Method of Journal Assertion and Manifestation

Manifestation works with the principle of the law of attraction. What you believe in strongly gets attracted to you! The 3-6-9 method is a proven way to assert yourself about what you feel and manifest it in the universe.

The method involves writing what you want to assert three times in the morning, six times at noon, and nine times in the evening. Nikola Tesla, a famous inventor, believed that these numbers are attributed to a great power in the universe.

Gather all your willpower to put your mind on what you need to assert. It can be about your health, happiness, strength of your mind, or anything you believe in. Once you do, you have to start practicing it. As you repeat yourself with the process, you will start observing the assertion vibing within yourself.

Kinship & Friendship - Roots to Happiness

At the end of your life, how much money you make doesn't count; it is the people you earn that matter. After all, what are you without family and friends! They are the only companions who stand all through your joy and pain. Life is not worth living long unless you have people you love around you. Don't you love a shared laugh or shared platter? Of course, you do! Hence it is vital that you make room for them in your everyday life.

Yes, I understand! Not every family is life. You don't get along with all the relatives. But at least there are few whom you cant create a connection with. However busy you are, ensure to allocate time for them! Laughing aloud is the greatest medicine! You cannot buy them alone. It is the friends that can make them happen. So, open your heart to them often.

72 Hour Rule - Master Control

Let it be friendship or love; every relationship goes through hard times. We make wrong choices when we are mad and angry. The words we say tend to cause irreversible damages and become a scar for a lifetime. If you desire a long, fulfilling life, trust me, you don't want to carry the baggage of guilt and regrets. So you need to get control of your emotions and reactions.

How am I supposed to control it?? Are you asking this yourself? Well, You have to use the 72-hour golden rule. As the name implies, do not react until 72 hours past the incident. Follow this rule strictly whenever you are angry and hurt. But why the 72 hours? It will give you enough time to sort out the situation. Anything can happen during this time. It might not even matter to you after 72 hours, or you might be ready to let go of it as it is not worthy of it. It is an effective way to get control of your emotions and reactions.

Mental health is an important aspect of quality life. So it is important to adhere to the healthy practices discussed in this chapter to travel in the road of long life. But the *12 rules journey* is not ending yet. We will be traveling in detail to the other rules in the upcoming chapters, so keep reading it.

Chapter 8: Live Long with a With a Healthy Lifestyle

Long-life comes not just by good diet and good health. It starts right from how you take care of your body daily and the kind of habits that occupy your day. Success depends on how well you organize your day and include the habits within your routine. Simply put, it is the lifestyle that determines your life span.

Have you ever observed your activities for a whole day? Do you utilize every minute of your day by doing productive activities? If your answer is "no" to both the questions, well, you are not alone. But since you are already here, worry no more. In this chapter, I will lay a framework for a healthy lifestyle. When you establish that in your life, you will be more than happy to answer the first two questions we came across at the start of this paragraph.

Health Management

Yes! We have already discussed healthy food, drinks, and mental health in the previous chapters. But why are we here again? Because we are digging deeper and will be delving into everyday practices. Even the way you walk, sit, and sleep affects your health in either a positive or a negative way.

Being cautious of what you do from morning to evening can noticeably improve your health. I pave the way for you to connect with this universe in the best way possible. We will dig into the long-forgotten tradition and practices that helped us thrive in the past. All the comfort and sophistication have taken us far away from Nature.

1. Work on Your Healthy Smile

When it comes to health, the most underrated is dental well-being. How many of us make regular visits to the dentist? Probably a minimal number! But I am talking here to even avoid the visit to the dentist. We brush in an automated way that we don't even realize that we are cleaning our teeth and mouth. So the next time you stand before the mirror to brush, pay attention to what you do. We have all learned about the directions and movement to brush effectively. So all you have to do is apply it correctly.

Minor additions to the usual routine are needed to make it perfect. Brushing is not just about your teeth but also about your tongue. So do remember to scrape your tongue. The consistent use of dental floss can keep it clean and wipe away the bacteria and plagues that might stay in your teeth from the food. Keeping the germs away will mean fending off the diseases and living healthily.

2. Utilize the power of Nature

Here at this moment, we live in a world where we reach even the farthest places with a touch of a button; we forget what we have at our doorstep. Hence, it is time to make the best use of whatever our Nature offers. Bringing yourself near to Nature and blending within is the secret to earning good health.

The feel of the ground under your barefeett is not only the nearness to Nature, but it can create a bond that can help you get the goodness of Nature. You can either call it earthing or grounding. You can even say it as part of preventive or alternative medicine. But it is just not the belief but science that the earth carries electrical charges on the surface. It is believed to possess anti-inflammatory properties that can benefit you. Hence make it a habit to walk barefooted every day for a while.

The Sun is perceived as a god all over the world. Many individuals and communities still start the day with a prayer to God. It is a known fact that the universe revolves around the sun. It is the elixir of life. Isn't it a shame to not utilize such power? Sunlight is a rich source of Vitamin D, vital for your bones. Hence, face the Sun and gain energy from the mighty sun. Try to look at the sun either during sunrise or sunset, when the heat intensity is low.

3. Daily Mandatory routine

A conscious and well-planned routine for the day can essentially affect your health. It is a discipline you insert into your lifestyle for longer life. Hence in this section, I put forth a few mandatory routines that you should follow without fail if you yearn to live long.

1. **Prayer** - It is important that you create time to do your prayer every day to have positive vibes in your life. If you are not a believer in God, you can use your creative visualization to positively impact your thoughts. It is a way in which you visualize what makes you happy. In turn, you enjoy the optimistic changes in your emotions.

2. **Oil Pulling** - Using edible oil such as coconut oil, clean your mouth by swishing it swiftly inside your mouth. The method is similar to mouthwash; you have to do it until the oil turns into a foam-like texture. It can keep the bacteria away from your mouth and acts as a detox for the body.

3. **Wall Posture** - If you want to live your long life proudly walking without any aid till the late years, you have to work on your posture. Wall posture straightens your spine and gives you a better walk. You might have been told that you are stooping your shoulders or your shoulders are not balanced. Wall posture straightens your spine and gives you a better walk. You can align it with this simple method. Lean against a wall by pressing

your head, shoulder blades, your butt, and keep your feet 2 or 4 inches away from the wall. Press the back of your palm on the wall behind the curve of your lower back. As you stand in this position, start walking, and do not forget to maintain it throughout the day.

4. **Mewing** - It is a simple method to have a better jawline. It is the process of placing your tongue in the right place. It is putting your tongue entirely in the upper part of the mouth while your tip of the tongue stays between the two front upper teeth.

5. **Chin Tucks** - Nowadays, most of your time is spent before the computer. Due to improper posture, many of you suffer from neck and shoulder pain. The head tuck or chin tuck exercise can strengthen your neck. Sit straight comfortably in a chair or wherever possible. Get your fingers to your chin and hold up your head while tucking it. Hold it as long as for a count of 5, release it, and bring it back to your finger. Repeat it at least ten times or till you can endure. Do it whenever possible in between your work every day.

6. **Door Frame Stretch** - Yet another exercise that can correct your rounded shoulders. Stand in front of any of the door frames in your house, and keep your hands on the door frame on either side. Align your hands to the length of the frame from elbow to fingers. Now push yourself forward as if you are going to walk into the

door. As you move to the front, you can get a stretch on the shoulders and hold it for at least 15 minutes. Repeat it 3 times to have a better effect.

7. **10 Minute rule for Toilet** - Toilet habits are more important for health management. The most important rule is to not sit in the bathroom for a long time while you don't feel you are done. Keep saying to yourself that you would never spend more than 10 minutes in the toilet. Avoid taking books and mobiles into the bathroom.

8. **Start with water** - Taking water on an empty stomach can help you with better digestion. Have a glass of water every day in the morning. It will kick-start your digestion journey for the day and energize you better by absorbing the minerals.

9. **Check Your Alignment**- As much as you concentrate on your posture, it is quite natural to forget the body alignment. As Katy Bowman says, you can check your posture by drawing lines after taking a picture of you while standing. Your shoulder, hip, and legs should be in a straight line.

10. **Watch Your legs While Driving** - If you are a person who travels a lot, you should pay attention to your posture while driving. It is important to have a good ergonomic posture to help you enhance efficiency and safety. Do not carry anything in your pocket while

driving; straighten up your spine, have a relaxed hand, and keep your feet flat on the car floor.

11. **Maintain Posture While Using Your Device** - Smartphones and mobiles have become an integral part of life. Let it be for entertainment or office communication; everything revolves around the mobile phone. Unfortunately, due to its convenience, we forget how and where we are sitting or lying. At the same time, we use it due to its convenience. Maximum posture issues start with the way you use your mobile. You are not allowed to drop your head or bend your neck to see the mobile screen. Such practices will lead to neck and spinal issues. Hence make sure the screen is in front of you whenever you are using the smartphone.

Routines and Aids to Make Your Lifestyle Better

A hassle-free life is a life that keeps you out of stress and anxiety. Hence it starts with having proper time management and financial management. Time and money are vital factors of life that are invaluable. Hence ensure you use it wisely.

Time management is all about planning everything before the event or need. It starts from keeping the things ready for tomorrow morning's cooking and materials for the meeting. A checklist is an efficient way to ensure you have everything in advance. The last-minute chaos is hard to handle, which adds to the stress.

A disturbed mind will sow the seeds to all kinds of diseases in the body. Hence you must stay in a clear mind each day. Take time to prepare a checklist for everything. It can be for both the household and the office. It is a one-time task; if you can create a template, you can easily use it every time. Once you establish the habit of preparing a checklist, you are likely to hold on to that habit forever. This is how you change a practice into a habit.

Whenever you are working, you can use the 20/20/20 rule to keep your eyesight and mental acuity sharp and fine. In an interval of 20 minutes, look away from your screen (laptop or mobile), and stare away for 20 seconds. You can choose anything that is 20 feet away from you to stare at.

Have a routine in your life that doesn't involve spending your maximum time on social media. It is a shame that nowadays, people who don't have time to talk with a friend spend all their time putting posts and status updates for the same friends and family. Isn't it funny?

Social media can be entertaining and relaxing, but only within the desired limits. It is known to ruin even relationships. Social media have the capacity to blind your real thoughts and influence you with uncertain information. You will be wondering to see the effect social media can have on your mind, and continuous use can affect your mind in an adverse way. Any adversity is a hindrance to health. Hence if you yearn for a long life, spend time in better ways like reading a book.

Music is the most desirable form of relaxation, and we all love to hear it. Be it at the home, workplace, while driving, or while traveling, we all keep hearing the songs. Are you one of those people who hear the songs in a way that it will be spilling out from the headphones? No. You shouldn't be. It can affect the hearing capacity during a long exposure. Your volume in a headphone should be at the level of someone near to you talking into your ears. It is the best way to hear the music you love.

Ayurveda, a natural system of medicine, originated in India more than 3,000 years ago. The term Ayurveda is derived from the Sanskrit words ayur (life) and veda (science or knowledge). Thus, Ayurveda translates to "knowledge of life". Ayurveda is best known for its alternative medicines. It also provides various objects that protect you from the negative energy floating around you. The metals such as copper and silver bracelets have a healing capacity as per ayurvedic medicine. The bracelets and crystals have positive vibrations in your body. Positivity creates healing and protection to the mind, body, and soul. The evil eye bracelets are perceived as protection from ill fate and negative things in your life. So make sure to wear one every day.

Yet another therapy that Ayurveda offers for creating assertion and strengthening your chi is the singing bowl. The music from the singing bowl penetrates the soul and creates an almost immediate bliss through your body. The tingling and the unusual calmness you get after you hear it has immense power. It ignites the core strength of your mind and soul. So make sure to hear it at least once a day.

Hence as we saw in this chapter, long-life is not about practice but a way of life you live. When you take care and pay attention to even the tiniest details in your day-to-day life, no one can take away the long life from you. The earth has so much to offer to you; it is only the effort to use it that is needed for an uninterrupted healthy life.

Daily life is not confined within your home and involves a daily life away from home. Until you figure out the way to keep yourself happy and stress-free in that environment, your daily life is not complete. But no worries, my ninth rule explains it in detail. It talks about having the right job and tackling the negativity of job-related life to live a long life.

Chapter 9: Loving Job: Strategy to ace the long-life game

The profession you choose plays an important part in your life. A job is where you will be spending the majority of your time in your complete lifetime. Hence, you cannot just choose any profession as your job. If you want to know you have landed the right job, ask yourself the following questions.

Do you feel excited to go to the office every morning? Does it give you the feeling of satisfaction and peace at the end of the day? Does the day usually go swiftly, or are you pushing your time through the day?

When you do a job that you love, you won't be stressed about it. Despite the hardships, you will keep enjoying every step of it and every moment. That is the kind of profession one should be doing. If not, it will become burdensome, and you will be carrying the weight in the mind and soul. Even if it offers you a fortune, a job should be something you love and do. Just doing it will make it meaningless.

If you are already enjoying it, all you have to do is keep doing it. If you are not, it is time you start looking for a change. It can look hard to switch jobs as you have your commitments and financial issues already going on in your life. But rest assured, all the inconvenience and hardships you will be going through to get the job you live in will be worth it in the end.

Once you land a job you love, you will start feeling at ease, and living it will be as easy as breathing. You will be doing your job as it is part of your life and not something you have to do by pushing yourself for it. Put your mind on the things you love; fame and money will follow it eventually. Hence you don't need to speculate over if you are making the right choice.

A long life needs a calm mind, strong thoughts, determination, and happiness. All this will be at stake if you cannot maintain a good habit at the workplace.

It is important to have a healthy lifestyle at home, it is equally important to follow the same in the office or job. Every moment of your life you live is yourself, and it affects you in a good or bad way with every happening. Hence, you can't ignore your lifestyle at your job, which forms the most significant part of your life.

As long as you stay happy and smiling all through your day, the long life will be near and dear to you. This chapter will detail the intelligent and efficient way to have a healthy lifestyle at your job. Follow the nine essential practices mentioned below in your work-life to introduce discipline in your work life. Following healthy habits is the paved road on which you travel towards a long life. Who wouldn't want to travel?

1. Find Balance and Stay Away from Stress

We already saw the importance of time management in the previous chapter. Hence, you should make sure to utilize the same discipline at the workplace. The time you spend at work should not be at the cost of your time with family and friends. It is important to stay true to yourself, but it is more important to have a happy mind. A happy mind has more potential than a coerced mind.

The next time you sit beyond your job time, think about whether this activity is critical enough to compromise your personal life? If it is important, you are bound to sit while working. Yet, think again! You sat there for an extra hour. Is it because it was unavoidable, or is it your mistake? Humans have the habit of carrying their work till the last minute until it becomes important. So, avoid such a last-minute rush and plan your day ahead. As long as you utilize every moment of the day productively, you will be amazed to see the time you save at work.

Stress and depression at work have a direct impact on the work-life balance. Think about it! You spend a long time toiling hard in your office. But there is no progress, no promotion, no incentives; it will be frustrating. But you cannot blame the employer entirely if you didn't plan your day properly. But if you think it is because of the workplace despite your planning, you should start thinking about whether you are in the right place. Money is important in life, but you should do a job you love rather than the job that pays.

2. Watch Your Food

When people are busy with their work at the office, they hardly notice what they eat. All the healthy recipes and food consciousness tend to disappear when you are at work. But no, it can't! Consistency should exist in life throughout the day. If not, you cannot really taste the benefits of long life.

It is time you start watching what you eat in your office. Just because you are busy and don't have much time doesn't mean you can slide down junk foods. Plan your meal ahead at your workplace so that you take only healthy foods, even at the office.

People bring all sorts of food to the office as a token of consideration to their colleagues. But that doesn't mean you have to consume all that unhealthy food to impress them. Having snacks in the afternoon can ruin your appetite and lead to overeating. Hence hop out of your office for lunch. Doing so will help you avoid snacks and give you a break from your work desk.

A desirable life needs a desirable job, and it comes with the satisfaction you get from your career. Such a feeling can happen when you can put forth 100% of your effort. But if you are sick often, can you show your full potential? Certainly not! That's why you need good eating habits even at the workplace. If you do, you can be consistent in your work and offer your best without health hindrances. It will create positivity within yourself and act as a motivation to stay happy every day.

3. Stay Away from Caffeine

A hot cup of coffee is all you crave when you are all stressed out at work. The moment you sip it, you might feel the mind easing. It will be so comfortable that you will lose track of the number of cups that went down your throat. Excess caffeine can negatively affect your gut health, so make sure to take only a minimal amount of coffee at work. If possible, try to count the number of coffees you drink at work. Knowing your intake might avoid excessive intake.

The caffeine might initially make you think like it's refreshing, and it is while it is within limits. The more caffeine you consume, the more you will be tempted to consume more. Hence it will be better to put it under control. The cravings will eventually lead to your ill health. It will disrupt your work and affect your efficiency.

4. Water is the elixir at work.

Mental work drains you more than physical work. Hence, you must drink enough water when you are working. When you are glued to your desk and the monitor, you will forget to sip the water. Hence try to keep a bottle of water next to you. You can avoid weakness and dizziness due to stress and strain at work if you are hydrated enough. If you think you could not drink much water, try having fruit juices in between work and meals.

5. Be Aware of Your Posture

While you are immersed in your work, it is quite natural to lose yourself and forget about yourself. When you are keenly watching your computer screen or while you are attending a meeting, you might absent-mindedly stoop to the front or cross your legs. This can affect your posture and put pressure on the spine, and will result in back pain. Hence remind yourself to sit straight with shoulders back whenever you are sitting in the chair.

The eye level is also an important factor while working with the laptop. The screen should be in straight alignment with your eyes. It should neither be above nor below your eye level; if it does, it will put pressure on your neck and cause pain. So make sure you have a proper table and chair that gives you the proper posture while working.

6. Make Sure to Move Around

The digital world has chained people to their chairs. So we suffer from many types of illness due to the tightening of muscles. So, why stress your body that way? Give it a movement now and then so that you can relax your body. Whenever you get a chance, make sure to walk a little. Even if you don't have the need, take a tiny break every 30 minutes to move your joints and body. Whenever you are at work, take the stairs instead of the lift. It will give the necessary movement to your knee joints.

7. Make Friends

Companionship is always desirable, and work buddies can make your office life much better. So try and get to know the people you are working with. You may have competition within your company, but a healthy friendship is not a hard thing to come by. All you have to do is be open to knowing them and making amicable connections with them.

If you can make friends at the workplace, you will always have ears to listen to and a shoulder to lean on. They can accompany you at lunch, and when you eat with a friend, you will be certain to take only healthy foods. If you are stressed, you can just bust it out on them, as they will understand you. In short, having a friendship at the workplace will be bliss as it will make the whole experience of working a lot better. If you are lucky enough, they can become your friend of a lifetime. Either way, you will see a positive aspect of having a good buddy at your job. So always make friends, and there is no limitation to making good companions.

8. Take time off

You might be so proud about how you have never taken any vacation and sincerely been there at the office, even during weekends. But is it something to prove your worth? Not really. No one is going to give you an incentive or an award just because you sacrificed your vacation for the sake of the work. Hence accept the fact that you deserve the time you take to spend it for yourself. So use all the days off given to you.

Even the employer and the rules know that productivity increases with proper rest. It is the reason why there is a separate leave allocation for vacations. Hence make sure to go on a vacation at least once a year. When you stay away from your work for a while, you will enjoy the change of scenery. A change like this always has a good impact on the mind. It will be like refreshing and revitalizing yourself. After this break, if you go back, you will feel more interested in your work and will put your 100% in your job. A calm mind can do big things, and quickly.

People witness heart diseases, stroke, cardiac arrest, and diabetes as early as in the late thirties. If you pile up all the studies together and analyze them, you will understand that most of them point towards stress. The worrisome medical condition for a human is stress. We never know in what way it will affect your life. Hence, it is important to clear out all the stress from your mind. Thus, the need for a vacation is evident.

The above lifestyle habits for the workplace are the strategy to ace the live long and long life game. Hence do not stop with reading it and start putting all these into action for a desirable outcome. Yes, a loving job is important! But having the right employer is also important. If you do not have a supervisor who cannot understand your basic human needs, then it is not the right place to work in. So you should ensure that you are in the right hands.

If you feel you are not comfortable working anywhere, you have the greatest choice of starting your own business. It can be risky, difficult, and full of hardships. But when you do it all for yourself, it will be more fundamentally rewarding. That is the positive side of having your own business.

Till this chapter, we saw the rules that will help you in the integral parts of life. As the foundation needs to be strong enough, we spent enough time seeing it to the tiniest detail. But it is time we go beyond your daily life that will keep you both healthy and happy. So keep reading to know about the other rules to enhance yourself.

Chapter 10: Living Long Needs a Passion for Happiness

Health, food, family, and job are an integral part of life; we care for them naturally. They are responsibilities, and they require our attention. But your duties do not make you complete. Yes! You find solace in your family time, health care, and profession. But is it enough for you? What do you do when you return from your job and feel tired of the routines? Despite having a lovely family and an amazing job, you are likely to face your down days.

Happiness is the only key to a long life. There is no alternative to your joy. I am not saying this with the mere aid of theory, but with the practical changes, we feel passion. It is your body's reaction when it feels joy and happiness. Now you know what having even a little joy can do to you!

Now, think about what if you can feel it every day? It will be an energy boost to your body and mind. Yes! You love to experience that and give your body an option to feel relaxed and be at ease. So how do we do that? It is pretty easy; find a passion that can keep you thriving. A passion can be anything from having a creative hobby or an outlet for your emotions. You might have a talent that is not related to your profession. You can still start pursuing it. You will be excited to accommodate time to follow your passion.

As long as it can make you feel delighted, it is worth making time out of your busy schedule. Yes! I know you are super busy juggling between work and family commitments. But you are the most important person to you in this world. This person needs special attention as well. If you believe in your ability, you are sure to accomplish time for passion.

You can love anything from as silly as collecting stamps to playing the cello. What's your passion? It doesn't matter; how much it can excite is what matters.

If you are right now wondering and struggling to think about your passion, do not worry. If watching a movie or listening to music delights you, it is also a passion. It can even be in the form of having a simple outlet for your mind. Still, are you confused about what your passion is? Do not worry; we will discover it

Know Your Passion

As I said earlier, happiness is vital to your stress-free life. Passion can make you indulge yourself with love and make you travel to a different world. It is also something that makes you do it no matter what. Hardships become negligible when you love something. If you already have one, it is good and well! But if you don't, it is time you start digging into what you like. In the upcoming section, I will help you identify your passion. So let us keep reading and travelling.

1. Look into What You Love

There might be hidden pleasures you always enjoy. But you might not realize how passionate you are about it. If you love something, you will feel the following.

- The urge to do it despite your busy schedule

- You will be drawn towards doing it without knowing

- It will fill you with happiness

- You will find yourself transitioning to a different world while doing it.

If you have felt all the above or any of the above, congrats, you already have your passion for pursuing. To make it real, you need to put more effort into it. You can explore more about your passion and make yourself better at it.

2. What Do You Research ?

But if you feel you can't find the one you love, ask yourself! Is there anything that you love to explore? While you look into the internet, what is the topic you often look for? When you have a passion or love something, you will unknowingly keep looking for it. Even if you don't look for it, the moment you come across it somewhere, you will be drawn to it. Suppose you have a keen interest in cooking but don't realize how passionate you are about it; You will be scrolling through all the new recipes trending on the internet.

Let's say you love gardening but never started it till now; you will find yourself ending up on google pages related to growing plants or knowing more about gardening. You will be curious to know about all the sales going on about the plants for growing in your backyard. Just because you have not started it yet, doesn't mean you don't have passion for it. Don't we all need a start for everything? Think of this as a start and change your interest into your passion. I am not trying to establish a skill for you here rather ignite the creativity in you.

Thinking in a new way utilizes the maximum capacity of your brain. It paves the way for healthy mind practices. Creativity helps you think in a fourth dimension and gives satisfaction to what you do. When you feel you have achieved something, happiness follows it.

3. Rack Your Brain

You have thought of everything, but you couldn't still land upon something that inspires you. Do not worry; I have got your back. We just need to dive deeper into your mind and life to sort it out. The best way to do it is to prepare a list. By pouring your mind, you will be able to know what you are passionate about.

Take a piece of paper and start writing the things you do or come across often. It can be playing chess, cooking, baking, gardening, looking for antiques, exploring new places, solving others problems, exploring different foods, soccer, decorating your home, volunteering, dancing, writing, and even financial investments. The above list are only examples, but it can be anything big or trivial, but it is important to you. Observe your daily routine and look around your house; it defines you better. From this, you will be able to identify what you like the most.

Always remember, it doesn't need to be something special or some unique talent to make it your passion. It can be a trivial thing like being curious about new movies or sharing your view on quora. Everything is talent in itself.

4. Ask a Friend

Suppose you find it difficult to identify a passion all by yourself; it is always good to have an outside opinion. Not everyone observes him/herself properly. It is, hence, better to have a third eye. But it has to be someone who has known you for a long time and has spent significant time with you. What are friends for? It is easier to ask them. They know you better!

So ask for an honest opinion about what you are good at in their eyes. You might be amazed by the answers you get. We have the habit of noticing other people's talents rather than ours. Hence, it is likely to come as an advantage to you.

I am sure that you will find your passion in any of the four ways mentioned above. So, now you are happy to know what your passion is. Next, what is the connection between your passion and a long life? I talked in detail and length about how to lead to your passion because it is something that gets you happiness despite all the tough situations.

When you experience joy and excitement, even your body understands it and responds accordingly. Even science supports the fact that people who are happy are less prone to diseases and chronic disorders. The reason why I am emphasizing passion is because it is not mentioned. Your school, college, family, and workplace are not gonna teach you the importance of doing what interests you.

Sometimes it is so hard that life doesn't come with a manual or instruction booklet. But my guide to the long life I am providing here will complement this need. I talked about a job, and now I am talking about a creative passion. Are you wondering what the difference is? Well, to put it simply, there are things we do for a need and things we do for our satisfaction. That is the precise difference between a job and a creative passion.

Money is a need, so you have to work. There are choices in a job as well; you get to choose your job of interest. But you cannot deny the fact that, be it a job or business, you have to compromise something to keep it afloat. But passion is something you do solely for the sake of your happiness. You do it because you like it and not because you earn money. It is also a way to put yourself ahead of others' needs. It can positively affect your health.

Why Do You Need to Have a Creative Passion?

I will explain why being happy is important, as happiness and passion are intertwined with each other. They help you live a rejoicing, long life.

Heart Health

Stress and tension can pile up and negatively affect health. We know what will happen to people who are under consistent mental pressure; they are prone to the risk of cardiac diseases. It is those days when we hear people getting heart attacks, even in the early 30s. So it is important that you pay attention to your emotions. Do you think people who are suffering from heart problems knew they were at risk? No. It was least expected. Stress has a way to penetrate your life, even without you knowing it.

A target pressure at office, disappointments over career growth, fights with loved ones and children, and anxiety of not being able to see growth. All of these create stress inside you without showing any signs. You presume that these are normal, and that is life. The moment you wake up the next day, you will be carrying on the same load all again. Hence, it is building pressure that has a huge impact on your heart. That is why you are supposed to vent out your stress. Sharing with people can reduce it, but it cannot make you forget it.

But when you have a passion, and you pursue it, you will lose your mind to it. Even if you cannot do anything, listening to a curated collection of songs will give you calmness in mind. It will give you moments where you will detach yourself from the current world. That is the beauty of being creative or keeping an outlet for yourself.

Enhances Immune System

Happiness is way more effective than any other medicine in the world. People who complain a lot, keep to themselves, and stress over little things are largely at the risk of falling sick. The people who open up, talk, and laugh a lot are more likely to have resistance to diseases than the grumpy people.

People with negative emotions are more vulnerable to the spread of diseases than happy ones. There are so many studies and literature supporting these facts. So it is visible evidence that happiness can keep you healthy enough to combat diseases. It conveys the message that you have a better immune system when you stay happy. But only along with healthy eating habits, as we discussed earlier in this book.

Hence, I insist on following up with your passion, even if you are busy with your full schedule. If we are to live long, we prefer a disease-free life.

Brings Down Stress

To rule out stress, you need to relax. It comes by doing something that can offer you happiness. People who always feel happiness and joy stay calm and composed even in stressful situations. Happiness can relax every cell in your body. Hence, happiness creates a calmness of mind and helps you combat every stress in your daily life.

Stress and happiness are not restricted to mental health but are intrinsically connected to the physiological health of the body. As we know, consistent exposure to stress can lead to physical conditions like ulcers, high blood pressure, and heart diseases; you should beware of your emotional state of mind. Ignoring your stress will only decrease the healthy lifespan of your precious life.

Passion can alter these mishappenings and can give you all the happiness you need. By being happy, you are staying out of mental turmoil, increasing the quality of your life. After all, a long life should be healthy and enjoyable. We will all agree on that!

Endurance to Pain

Happy people are stronger than those who are not. When you are happy, you are more assertive, and you won't be shattered that easily. Be it a mental burden or physical stress; you can face it better than anyone else if you are prone to consistent happiness. Even among patients who are going through chronic diseases and facing pain often, the happy ones fight the illness a lot better.

Hence you can say that the happiness in your life pours you with positivity and helps you develop strength mentally and physically. When you are that strong, no pain can break your trust in life. You should be able to fight every adverse moment with a smiling face if you are to live a long life.

So, I can point out many examples to prove the fact that joy is inevitable if you are aiming to live long. They are not mere myths but scientifically proven facts. Now you can understand why I emphasize the need to have a passion. As the sun is to the solar system, the passion is for a healthy life.

Chapter 11: Belief in a Higher Power

Spirituality to a person is not a religion but a belief. What is the purpose of life without beliefs? Have you ever trusted something that you cannot see but only feel?

Those questions were not for you to answer but to reflect on yourself. You can belong to any religion, any ethnicity, or you can even be an atheist; belief helps you cross the dire straits. When you are put in a critical situation, you tend to test your capability to do better. All of a sudden, why were you able to do it? Because you believed and put the burden on an unknown power, and you did it. That is the beauty of having a belief.

To put it simply, it is a relationship that goes beyond the materialistic connections and is attached to your soul. There are no defined rules for pursuing spirituality. As long as you have trust, nothing else matters. It can be the customs, prayer, community rituals for a few, and for a few others, it might be silence, meditation, and detachment from the world; that can mean spirituality.

Spirituality can go beyond solving mental stress. When the body is going through physiological strain, the mental state of mind will be naturally affected. When you have belief, it can help you fight the adverse effect on the body by easing your mind. You would have noticed your mind seeking the help of the ultimate power when going through the worst times. It is because you trust that the superior power will listen to you and help you out of the situation.

Can you live a life that doesn't have any meaning at all? No, you cannot. Life will be monotonous, and you will be bored. Whenever life hits rock-bottom, you need an anchor to hold on to life. If not, you will more likely give up. Your dream for a long life will be shattered into pieces.

As I mentioned earlier, there is more than one way to establish spiritual practices in your life. The methods I enlist here will be for everyone. Starting from the devout believer to the atheist, everyone can follow my ideas as long as they have a belief in them.

Mind-Body Practices for Health Control

Contemplative practices mean having control over one's thoughts and awareness flowing inside and outside one's soul and body. In simple terms, those are practices that make you aware of your mind and body. They have deep roots in the tradition, and there are different ways to follow it. Why do we need to do it? It keeps your mind alert, conscious, wide-awake, focused, confusion-free, and calm. Such a strong mind can wear away any kind of negative and depressing thoughts and stay undisturbed by them.

A mind that can control its thoughts and master the art of contemplation is the strongest. They are filled with positive thoughts like empathy, kindness, and concentration. A sturdy mind is needed for a long life. Hence creating a routine to practice spirituality should be the eleventh rule of your long-living journey. We will see the methods of contemplation that you can follow to practice the same.

As I already mentioned, spirituality is a belief rather than a connection to religion. Hence, whatever religion you are, whatever beliefs you have, you can still follow all these practices in your daily life.

1. Meditation

It needs only five minutes of your day for meditation, and it will significantly improve your mental health. It will reinforce positive thoughts. Science, with the aid of researchers like Richard Davidson, has put forth evidence for the fact that meditation can enhance the betterment of gray matter in the brain. It helps the brain to combat your body's complex emotions and feelings.

Mindfulness is one way of meditation in which you establish control over your thoughts. The pain and complex emotions become less difficult to handle when you practice meditation. Once you practice daily, you will gain control over the thoughts that make you anxious. This, in return, has a greater impact on the body, like reducing the risk of type 2 diabetes, chronic pain and fatigue, depression, rheumatoid arthritis, and cardiovascular disease.

2. Prayers

Prayers are done with the belief that there is the existence of an ultimate power watching over us. Our prayers convey our trust that the invisible savior will guide us to avoid ruin. During difficult times we call on them with the hope that our words will be heard.

Practicing prayers at the start and end of the day can be an optimistic reinforcing habit. Prayers have the power to imbibe positive force in your mind, and positivity of thoughts can induce improvement in body health. Do you need to choose a religion or God to do this? No. All you need is trust in the superior force that has control over this universe. If you are already a believer or a member of a certain religion, you can follow those customs regarding prayer. What matters, in the end, is creating the habit.

3. Yoga

We saw the importance of yoga in previous chapters as well, and here we connect it to the spiritual well-being of the mind. Contemplation includes all the practices that can control and streamline the thoughts of your mind. When practiced in the right way, yoga creates a free flow of thoughts inside your soul and keeps you relaxed.

It establishes the union of mind, body, and thoughts. If you had observed keenly, the movements of yoga demand a high level of concentration, attention, endurance, and stability. If you can establish all these in your life, the core of your mind becomes indestructible. Even the darkest thoughts cannot disturb you in any way.

4. Journals

Journals have the power of manifestation. Writing is one underrated practice that can positively impact your mind. To practice contemplation and have control over your thoughts, you should connect with the inner you. Journaling can create this connection for you.

I would recommend you to write at least one sentence a day. This can be a positive thought or a wish you would want to happen. Especially writing what cannot be achieved by yourself will give you the strength and belief to try beyond the possibility. It creates the resilience to bounce back swiftly during adverse conditions.

These four ways discussed above are effective ways to contemplate. It creates a strong habit that helps you to survive both through the day and in life. It is the best-laid foundation for a healthy and long life ahead.

Become Part of a Community

Would it be fun to celebrate your birthday or wedding party alone? No. Because there is no happiness alone. Friends and family are the people who make it a special moment. Similarly, spirituality is best savored in the group. You might have belief over different things, yet a community waits for you outside.

Try to locate a community that has similar beliefs as you do. And join with them to enjoy your spiritual journey. Attending mass prayers, group yoga, and meditation sessions can improve mental well-being. A regular habit of visiting such a community gives trust, security, and a feeling of motivation in your life.

Combat Hardships in Better Way

The trauma we face in our life makes it difficult to bring it back to normal. It takes quite a lot of determination and consequences to come through those periods. But people who believed in spirituality were stronger and more resilient to such situations. When you are at your lowest, you need the best kind of support you can get. But traumatic situations are complicated.

People who have gone through major incidents in their life like war, abduction, and confinement will not get along with people. They are stressed, curled in, and afraid. They do not prefer to contact people and do not wish to share their stories with anybody. The trauma will leave them in shock, guilt, self-pity, shame, and fear. We should give them time and an empathetic ear.

All the four methods we discussed earlier in this chapter for contemplation are effective, and you can make your pick. It will help you find purpose and realization of such difficult situations. But it needs trust in the power above to heal through the process. People who follow spirituality and inculcate such habits in their lives have a better vision to take even the traumatic situation as a chance to mold themselves. They see that as the opportunity to shape themselves into a better person.

After all, life is not filled with rosy paths! It is obvious that a road that has ups will certainly have downs. The more you accept, the easier it will be for your to bounce-back. We all know that people around us go through way more hardships than we. But the mind doesn't accept it easily, and it toils in self-pity. Spiritual practices help you understand and create acceptance of such hard truth.

Make the Right Choices

As you start practicing spirituality, you will create values and a vision for yourself in your life. The religions or beliefs have a layout containing rules. It also gives options for having a healthy sustained life. Everybody doesn't need to adhere to every rule put forth by the religion, but you can follow the one that suits you. There are people who have forsaken the consumption of meat after they started believing in spirituality. Since they believe such sacrifice can bring them a better life, we make the right choices. It is one such example, and there are many to go.

A calm mind can think right even in a stressful situation. We have all gone through that. When anger, fear, and frustration are at their peak, we make decisions and talk words that we regret forever. Don't we all make that mistake? But when you adopt spirituality, you are sure to be in a state of sanity all through the day. Hence, it will help you stay calm, look into the situations, and act accordingly. When you live a life where there are no regrets, it will be the best way to live a life. When there is nothing to worry about, happiness surrounds you and increases your lifespan.

Forgiveness is a Virtue

Hatred is a strong negative feeling that can bring down both your body's psychological and physiological health. But spirituality guides you on the right path and helps you to stay away from such pessimistic thoughts and behavior. It trains the body to sort and reason with the situations. It especially helps you to accept things.

You cannot live a healthy life by holding a grudge against someone. Negative thoughts are intense and feed on your energy. But love can heal even your sour soul and mind. Hence, start believing. If a child doesn't trust that it cannot walk, it will never walk in its lifetime. But what makes it walk without fear? Does it put trust in the mother and father?

The child knows the mom and dad are there to hold on to it and will never let it fall down. That's the kind of belief that will help us to overcome any hard situation. You will realize that nothing good will come out of being mad at someone for a long time. So start forgiving people, accept their ignorance, and move on quickly.

Spirituality is real, it is science, and it is a fact. So it is not a superficial thing I am talking about here. But proven facts. If you dive into literature, you can see vast studies proving the fact that spirituality increases a man's life. There are stories of yogis in the past and present living a long life. How did that happen? They do not possess any superpower. But they keep themselves poised and balanced. The worldly emotions don't shatter them, and they do not have expectations from the people of the society. They blend themselves with nature and live what it offers to them.

But I am not proposing you become a yogi but a believer. It is the secret ingredient to a calm and long life.

So spirituality is an aid to detach yourself from all the negative aspects of life. Even people who were drug addicts and drunkards have found solace in spirituality. They took this path to come out of this adverse life they live in. This chapter gave a glimpse of the benefits you reap if you follow the eleventh rule. I would say it is the easiest to follow but gives maximum benefit. So the ball is in your court and waiting for you to make the winning move.

Chapter 12: Dopamine Fasting to Have a Productive and Longer Life

Your mind is smart enough to trick you! The way the brain works and its physiological reaction in the body has a lot to do with your ability and productivity. What your eyes see sends the message to your mind, and it sends specific instructions to the rest of your mind as a reaction to the stimuli. Yes! It is a known fact. But the pleasure center of the brain can be quite complicated and addictive.

When you indulge yourself in social media, let us say watching TikTok videos, favorite web series, or merely scrolling through the posts of people, it reaches the brain, which in turn produces dopamine, a neurotransmitter. Once your body enjoys it, there is a high possibility of your getting addicted to it. You will be intrigued to do the things that create dopamine in your body. If you have always wondered why you are glued to your mobile and how hard you try to stay away, this is your answer. It is a dopamine addiction.

If you yield to these needs, you will waste tons of time in your life. Productivity will go to rock bottom if you cannot control it. So in this chapter, I will help you understand more about this dopamine detox and explain why and how you should do it. So keep reading to make use of your time in a better way. We will start from point zero!

What is Dopamine Detox?

Dopamine detox is keeping yourself from pleasurable activities like sugar consumption, scanning the social media or digital platforms, or unlimited shopping. These are not activities that are bad if done once in a while. But our body plays the trick by giving the feel of pleasure whenever we do such things that excite us. It lured us into doing it again and again as it saw the taste of it.

On the contrary, life's important and vital activities like studying, doing chores, and working don't give us pleasure. We find it boring and monotonous; we don't feel rewarded. Sitting in the classroom listening to complex equations, attending long meetings on a tiring day, or doing unending chores, none of these are even good for imagination, right? But why? It is because we don't secrete dopamine during these activities.

What happens when you get used to the dopamine of the body? You will lose control of what you do and will be drawn towards pleasure-giving activities. It is no different from drug addiction or alcohol addiction. Can you imagine yourself wasting your time and health over guilt pleasure and living the rest of your life regretting it? Certainly not. It is not the picture of a fulfilling life, so we will not do that.

These dopamine-seeking activities are impulsive in nature. How often do you toss your mobile, deciding not to see it and be back to it within an hour? It is because you are doing it without even realizing it. Before you even come to your senses, you have already spent considerable time in it. The most common impulsive practices are

1. Shopping

2. Gambling

3. Adventure-seeking

4. Pleasure or stress eating

5. Digital use

6. Games

Those mentioned above are the primary activities that can happen without our control. If unnoticed, they have the capacity to ruin health and relationships. Hence you cannot let it happen to you.

I propose dopamine detox as the way to refine your life and get you back on track whenever you feel like you lost it. Detox, as the name suggests, is a method to purify your thoughts and body. Like the detox water that cleanses your body by kick-starting your metabolism, dopamine detox cleanses the dopamine secretion from your body. The normalization will happen only when the body again realizes how it is to be without that impact.

How to do Dopamine Detox?

Before you start your dopamine detox, you should know what activities refrain you from being productive throughout the day. You can make a note of those. But you should also know that there has to be some amount of dopamine in your system to keep it balanced. Here I am not, hence, implying that dopamine is bad.

So let us dive into doing the dopamine detox. Choose any one day of the week that you are comfortable with. Stop doing things that you felt like pleasure-yielding activities. You will go through a cleansing process. But it is only for your brain, and you will be depriving yourself of all the pleasure. The purpose is to make your mind a clean slate. When you start from zero, your mind will start understanding what is important.

Dopamine addiction is similar to staying in a hallucination, and they cloud our mind from thinking straight. You eventually start listening to the cravings because your mind got used to the pleasure it gave you. So when you follow detox, it will break this unreal feeling, and you will be in reality. When the mind understands the importance of an activity, it will start loving even the boring things. When you know you are going to enjoy the clean house, you will enjoy doing chores. An A grade result will make the classes more interesting.

We all know the importance, but the pleasure we enjoy due to dopamine shields the facts. We act impulsively without even reasoning just to get the fix. So if you are to stay focused, stay on track with your life progress, keep your health in check, then follow the one-day-per-week dopamine detox routine without fail.

Why Should You Do Dopamine Detox?

Dopamine is not just related to how you feel your pleasure. The science behind it is so large that I can write a separate book for it! So let us say it is a chemical messenger of the body that communicates between two nerve cells. From the brain, it travels to other parts of the body. It lets the human mind do special things like think, find, seek, focus, and plan.

The connection goes beyond just your mind, but it has an influence over behavioral and physical activities.

1. Movement

2. Focus

3. Lactation

4. Pain control

5. Nausea and vomit control

6. Functioning of blood vessel

7. Functioning in kidney

8. Heart rate

9. Motivation

10. Mood

11. Sleep

So it explains why the long live rule talks about the dopamine detox. It is connected to all sorts of activities in your body; if imbalanced it will lead to interruption in your daily life. So it is right to say that just like your body's metabolism, the brain also needs kick-starting now and then.

Mental health is dependent on mood, motivation, and focus, which makes the role of dopamine inevitable. Even the reduced dopamine level of the body can have adverse effects such as poor alertness, less concentration, sluggishness and lack of happiness, clumsy coordination.

You should not fill yourself with euphoria or deprive yourself completely of it. Hence we should work on dopamine detox with 100% involvement.

1. Break the Comfort

The fluffiness of the sofa, with laptop in your lap, the juices and snacks scattered around you, and endless time scrolling the social media pages! How often do you see yourself in such a situation? Maybe quite often! Who can be blamed! It is such a bliss to spend time like that.

You are naturally inclined towards doing it again and again. Yeah! Your chores are pending, and your books are waiting for you to open! But who wants to do such boring things when you can laze around in the comfort of social media. This is the exact situation happening in your mind.

Will a child listen if you tell him not to eat the candy after letting him taste it? Of course not! In fact, he will do all kinds of tantrums to get the candy. It is the dopamine doing! This is why you have to break this ongoing cycle now and then to remind yourself that comfort is not going to make your life any better.

2. Get Your Thinking Ahead

The temporary euphoria of the dopamine effect blinds you from thinking on a long-term basis. It only lets you concentrate on the immediate pleasure and comfort you get through its effect. That is why you deviate from your path of productivity and creativity. The diversion can nullify all the efforts you have put in your life to be where you are.

Imagine this! You have not been this addicted from the day you were born! Maybe you were quite active till six months back. Now measure how much you have lost by being addicted to those things which gave you literally nothing in your life. If you keep a log of the time you spent devouring the pleasures, you will be shocked!

The detox can cleanse your mind and give you further vision. When you can perceive the long-term effects of whatever you are doing, you are sure to make only the right decisions. Better thinking gives you a better lifestyle, which will lead to a longer life.

3. Expand Your Vision Out of the Box

Only a clear and calm mind can allow creativity from within. Dopamine detox wears away the influence of pleasure and enables better thinking. When you get creative, you get passionate about life. Eventually, you will become your own love, and you will remain young by heart. People who smile often seem to stay longer for a long time. Hence I mentioned earlier; happiness is the crucial component of life.

Think of the days of our parents or even better of our grandparents. Communication technology was at its primitive stage; they naturally had less distractions in their lives. They weren't perfect, but they had a healthier lifestyle than we did because of the lack of high-tech devices. They didn't enjoy the comforts we have now; even if they had, it was a luxury and rare. You can still see our grandparents walk with the straight spine in their 90s!! Isn't it amazing? Dopamine detox is a way to relive those days.

Like any addiction, the dopamine detox may not be easy to tackle. Initially, it will be tough. If you believe and trust yourself, you will accomplish it. If you think you want motivation, do it along with a friend. Or, if you want self-motivation, you can do the detox in an alternative way. Thinking about your perfect life, finishing your chores on time, submitting assignments promptly, and when you receive appreciation from your boss for the extraordinary work, will help you sustain the detox process.

Instead of doing it one time a week, you can have an alternative cycle of three and one. For every three days of successful dopamine detox completion, you can treat yourself with those cravings for one day. This keeps you eager to do it and endure it. As the cycle goes, you will be happy to see how much you can increase the cycle gap. Eventually, you will bring balance to the dopamine level in the body.

Conclusion

We come to live this life with an empty canvas. Our intentions, aspirations, lifestyle, understanding, and practices are the elements that make it beautiful or ugly. We are all born with the talent and opportunity to fashion our life into beautiful art. But do we really appreciate it?

When the world fell into the pandemic, it saw innumerable deaths, which was disheartening! The lives of people I came across and those who lived around me made me think. Is life that hard? Why all that suffering? While we all were in this crisis together, why do some have to go, while others survive? Still, many of us are alive here today because of sheer luck.

What went wrong then? It is our ignorance. When we had it all, we didn't respect it. So, what is the "it" here? It is everything: food, money, jobs, lifestyle, beliefs, nature, and more. The moment the shops closed their doors during the pandemic, we learned how to optimize our resources. Many of us went into isolation, and we rushed into healthy eating. Companies around the world started shutting down, and people lost their jobs. To the people who were still at a job, it became dear to them. We weren't supposed to leave the house; family time became a boon.

The happenings of my life events inspired me to share the knowledge I gained through the years. Hence, I am here telling you my twelve rules secret of long life to you. In a life where we are running behind our jobs and daily routine, we forget what is important. How many of us are actually conscious about what we are eating? We grab it on the go to the office, or we absent-mindedly eat it while forgetting ourselves on our mobile.

But the first rule of this book explained to you why what we eat matters. I didn't stop by just telling you that but have provided you with a complete guide with the dos and don'ts to your diet. As it is the foundation for your health, I have given as much information as possible.

The first step to change is always hard; there will be no stopping once you go past it. So you better start eating healthy. You will see the significant change almost instantly as you start using the guide. When we talk about health, it is not just the food but also the proper liquid intake that matters to you.

Hydration of the body is the best way to flush out all the bacteria and germs. Water is also the source of energy for the body. If you are deprived of proper fluids in the body, you will feel weak all the time. Without proper hydration, you will be inviting all kinds of diseases to you. Hence the second rule helps you know beyond water. There are so many health drinks that can make you rejuvenate and feel new. The key is information, and I have given you access to that. Now it is your turn by following the second rule to stay healthy.

Mother nature has blessed us with everything humans need to survive in this world. Even before technology and science came into place, people survived every kind of crisis. It is because they had an intimate relationship with nature. The ancestors depended on nature but not on mankind for their survival. They utilized the riches of nature in the best way. The medicinal plants were long-forgotten as we shifted to sophisticated medicines.

Hence, as the third rule for long life, I have shared my detailed knowledge on some useful herbs that come in handy in our day-to-day lives. By adding these herbs to your routine, you will take your health to the next level. All the drinks might not suit everyone, so you can choose the one that makes you comfortable.

A healthy body cannot make life successful. Whom you keep around has a major impact on the quality of your life. That makes family and friends an integral part of us. The journey of life has no meaning if you do not have people to share with, lean on, and shower your love with. The fourth rule guides you through why and how you should be spending your time with family. It is not the quantity of time but the quality of time you spend for them that matters. If you have a shoulder to cry on, a hand to hold on to, and a heart to listen to, you can have a complete life.

Do you know the quality of your sleep can determine the kind of life you are living? Only a rested mind can beget calmness and the strength to live in this world. Deprivation of sleep will hinder your health despite healthy eating. So make sure to grab a good sleep every night to ensure you reap the benefits of good health. Your sleeping pattern also determines how good your day will be! Would that be a good day if you had not slept enough? I don't think so! You will feel sluggish and tired the whole day. Only a good sleep gives you a fresh start! So don't forget to follow the fifth rule! Next is sustaining the health you have created through good eating habits. Health is built with food, but strength comes with exercise. Hence make sure to stretch your body every day!

The seventh rule is about your mental health. A sound mind makes a healthy soul. What you feel within reflects on the outside. If having a strong personality is your desire, then certainly, you need to work on your mental health. As long as you have proper guidance, you can achieve it. This book has everything you want to know, hence make the best use of it.

The eighth and ninth rules of a healthy life are important to building your life. From food to mental health, we saw the separate components that are vital to life. But lifestyle is where you assemble these into habits. You make it a way of living that your life and these rules will become one and the same. Similarly, the job you do has a great contribution to this lifestyle. Hence, the choice you make is important.

The last three rules are reinforcing factors of your long life. The supporting factors such as passion, spirituality, and Dopamine detox help you to keep yourself together through the tough times of your valuable life.

I gained incredible pleasure in my journey with you all through this book. My success is not when you buy this book, but when you all follow these twelve rules to live a long life!!

Bibliography

American Bible Society (2010). *Holy Bible : Containing the Old and New Testaments : King James Version*. New York: American Bible Society.

Becker, A. (2016). *The 10 pillars of wealth : mind-sets of the world's richest people*. Dallas, Tx: Brown Books Pub Group.

Bet-David, P. (2021). *YOUR NEXT FIVE MOVES : master the art of business strategy*. S.L.: Gallery Books.

Covey, S.R. (2014). *The 7 habits of highly effective people : powerful lessons in personal change*. New York: Simon & Schuster.

Dalio, R., 2018. *Principles*. Simon and Schuster.

Ehret, A., 2012. *Mucusless Diet Healing System: Scientific Method of Eating Your Way to Health*. Book Publishing Company.

Ehret, A., 2012. *Rational Fasting: For Physical, Mental, and Spiritual Rejuvenation*. Book Publishing Company.

Fosse, L. (n.d.).
Bhagavad Gita The Original Sanskrit and An English Translation. [online] Available at:
https://library.um.edu.mo/ebooks/b17771201.pdf.

Greene, R., 2000. *The 48 laws of power*. Penguin.

Jethro Kloss (2011). *Back to Eden : a human interest story of health and restoration to be found in herb, root, and bark*. Whitefish, Mt: Literary Licensing Llc.

Maroon, Joseph M.D. (2008) *The Longevity Factor: How Resveratrol and Red Wine Activate Genes for a Longer and Healthier Life*. Simon and Schuster.

Maulawi Sher Ali (2009). The Holy Quran - Arabic Text w/ English Translation. [online] Available at: https://www.alislam.org/quran/Holy-Quran-English.pdf.

Myss, C.M. and Myss, C., 1998. *Why People Do Not Heal and how They Can*. Harmony.

Ober, C., Sinatra, S.T. and Zucker, M., 2010. Earthing: The Most Important Health Discovery Ever?. Basic Health Publications, Inc..

Passman, D.S. (2020). *All You Need To Know About The Music Business*. 10th ed. S.L.: Simon & Schuster.

Raylee, K., Wader, T., Claire, S., Michael, D. and Shaw, T., What Others Are Saying about the Writings of Professor Spira.

Ruiz, M., Jose Luis Ruiz and Mills, J. (2011). *The fifth agreement : a practical guide to self-mastery*. San Rafael, Calif.: Amber-Allen.

50 Cent, (Musician and Greene, R. (2013). *The 50th law*. London: Profile Books.

William, A. (2020). *Medical medium cleanse to heal : healing plans for sufferers of anxiety, depression, acne, eczema, lyme, gut problems, brain fog, weight issues, migraines, bloating, vertigo, psoriasis, cysts, fatigue, pcos, fibroids, uti, endometriosis & autoimmune*. Carlsbad, California: Hay House, Inc.

Made in the USA
Coppell, TX
20 May 2022

77993994R10085